"A formidable book. Essential reading for anyone
who wants to make sense of the biggest political
scandal in recent memory."
– Carol Vorderman

"Russell Scott has produced the definitive no-holds-barred
account of the biggest public-spending scandal in a generation.
Forensic, meticulous, packed full of incredible examples of
cronyism and corruption. Essential reading"
Peter Geoghegan

First Edition

VIP Lane

Cronyism and the pandemic

By Russell Scott

London, United Kingdom

Byline Books
London, United Kingdom

First published in the United Kingdom of Great Britain and
Northern Ireland by Byline Books, 2025

Cover Design by Mecob

Layout by Prepare to Publish

Printed in Great Britain by Clays

ISBN UK: 978-1-916754-16-4

For Harriet, Frances and Finn

Contents

Preface

There is a growing narrative in the UK that all politicians are cut from the same cloth and the political parties they are affiliated with cannot be trusted to be honest. A recent survey found that 58% of those surveyed in the UK "almost never" trust our MPs to tell the truth when in a "tight corner" – a 22% increase since the Covid-19 pandemic started.[1]

Shortly after taking power, the new Labour government found itself in the centre of a political storm over the PM Keir Starmer's vulnerability to accepting free hospitality in the form of Premier League football matches and tickets to see Taylor Swift's sell-out world tour.

I do not intend to downplay the public anger over the MPs accepting thousands of pounds' worth of freebies, especially as the vast majority of us are still feeling the pinch of this country's never-ending austerity drive. However, to understand the reason for the sharp fall in confidence in our political system over the past few years, one needs to take a step back from 'Swiftgate', rewind the clocks to 2020 and examine closely the previous Conservative Party government's response to the

Covid pandemic and the industrial-scale cronyism and political scandals that consumed the then PM Boris Johnson's time in No. 10.

Between March 2020 and March 2022, the UK government spent £311 billion on "pandemic-related support measures". The equivalent of handing £4,631 to every person in the UK, that figure could rise to as much as £373 billion, according to the National Audit Office.[2]

A staggering £96.7 billion was spent by the Department of Social Care (DHSC), which led on the flagship vaccination, PPE and Test and Trace programmes. At least £15 billion was wasted procuring goods from dubious sources – often purchasing products that were not fit for purpose and excessively inflated in price. That £15 billion wasted on unusable equipment could pay the annual salary of 441,000 NHS nurses.

The government established a 'VIP lane' that allowed companies with direct links to the ruling Conservative Party to jump the queue and land government contracts valued in the billions of pounds to provide medical equipment. The UK was the only nation in the world to introduce such a controversial and unlawful back channel during the pandemic.[3]

The government, under Rishi Sunak's watch, made the decision to incinerate billions of items of unusable PPE and to date, no VIP lane companies have been found guilty of any criminal wrongdoing or faced the consequences of plundering vast sums from the public purse – a track record that continues to anger many.

Millions of Brits are now grappling with the financial pressures of the current 'cost of living' crisis. Many are struggling to pay their mortgages, rent, bills and groceries – a striking juxtaposition when compared to the individuals who grossly profited from the government's unlawful VIP lane. These individuals are now splashing the cash on private jets, super yachts, stately homes and luxurious villas – a position many of the VIP lane recipients found themselves in not by merit, but because of the political connections they had within the governing Conservative Party.[4]

A reported 227,000 people died in the UK as a result of Covid-19. Heroic NHS front-line staff routinely went into battle against an unknown virus, putting their health on the line to protect our loved ones – often without adequate PPE to keep them safe. Many paid the ultimate price, a fact that shouldn't be forgotten when we also talk about the cronyism that overshadowed the government during a crucial moment in our history.

This book hopes to provide some justice to the people who gave everything to keep us safe.

Introduction

If somebody told me back in early 2020 that I would be writing a book today about government cronyism that centres around the procurement of personal protective equipment (PPE) or novel testing kits bought during a global pandemic, I would have thought they were slightly crazy.

But here I am, four years later, typing away and reflecting on a mind-boggling period of time that changed not just my life, but everybody's life in one eventful way or another.

Coronavirus, Covid-19 or simply Covid, an infectious disease caused by the SARS-CoV-2 virus, has taken on many labels since it first hit the news in January 2020 following an outbreak in the city of Wuhan, the capital city of Hubei Province in the People's Republic of China.

I still vividly remember being glued to BBC News, refreshing its home page every ten minutes and anxiously scrolling through my Twitter feed (or X as it's now called) in January and February watching the virus creep closer to our shores.

By late February 2020 the anxiety was almost unbearable

as country after country entered various forms of lockdown – 'lockdown' being a term that pre-pandemic I had never heard of, but one that came to dominate all of our daily discussion throughout 2020 and into 2021 as we grappled to come to terms with our new normal.

In late February 2020, the Lombardy region of northern Italy was becoming overwhelmed by a surge in coronavirus cases, labelled the worst outbreak of the virus in Europe at this point in time. Italian authorities decided to enforce a lockdown on 11 towns across the region. Surreal images emerged depicting empty roads, deserted pavements, shops boarded shut, squares devoid of people as the virus ravaged the district. At that point, 229 cases had been reported in the region and seven people had died. Italy eventually entered into a national lockdown on 9 March 2020. Controversially, Boris Johnson, the UK's newly elected prime minister, decided he would forge a different path for this country and held back on imposing a lockdown of any sorts. Instead, during a press conference on 3 March 2020 he gleefully boasted about a recent hospital visit where he shook everybody's hands, including some patients who had contracted the virus – unsurprisingly three weeks later Mr Johnson announced he had tested positive for Covid-19.[1][2]

By mid-March 2020, France, Spain, Belgium and Switzerland had followed Italy's path as country after country started to implement national lockdowns in a desperate attempt to slow down the spread of the virus and protect their citizens. The UK government remained slow off the mark, an outrider – seemingly distracted by other issues, notably Brexit and the country's difficult exit from the European Union. Far from closing down the country, 60,000 people were allowed to attend the Cheltenham Festival, crowds packed in tightly in the stands to watch the Gold Cup as the virus ripped through Europe.[3]

By 16 March, there was still no national lockdown. Instead Boris Johnson went on television and urged the British public to avoid all "non-essential contact" but seemingly ignored his own advice three days later to hold a "personal" meeting with influential Russian oligarch Evgeny Lebedev. Dominic Cummings, the PM's advisor at the time, would later claim in his witness statement issued to the Covid Inquiry that the pair discussed the Russian's future peerage during the 19 March meeting. This alleged meeting would typify Boris Johnson's lacklustre response and respect for following the rules. His constant contradictions were his modus operandi and in many ways defined his premiership during the pandemic.[4][5]

Finally, on 23 March 2020, a date permanently etched in many of our brains, the UK entered its first nationwide lockdown. By now 5,687 people had tested positive for Covid and 281 people had lost their lives from the virus. Boris Johnson sat behind his desk, with his trademark scruffy blond locks and a Union Jack flag hanging behind his left shoulder as he addressed the nation. The PM announced that with immediate effect shops selling non-essential goods would close. Libraries, playgrounds, gyms and places of worship were also shut. All gatherings of more than two people in public were prohibited. Weddings, baptisms and all social events were cancelled. Johnson ended this historic speech by enlisting the nation to "join together to halt the spread of this disease". He concluded with a slogan that would define the drumbeat of our lives for months to come: "Stay at home, protect our NHS and save lives".[6][7]

Journalism until this point was a part-time role for me. I was still finding my feet in a tough industry following a recent career change. Suddenly in between commissions I found myself juggling mortgage holidays and universal credit applications as my wife and I desperately tried to stretch the little savings we had squirrelled away for a rainy day or, in this case, a pandemic.

My launch pad into Covid-linked investigations didn't start where you'd expect. In April and May 2020, I hadn't yet picked up the trail of crony contracts or politically linked PPE suppliers, although I had heard murmurings from sources that all wasn't well inside the Department of Health and Social Care (DHSC). Instead, my focus was on pangolins – a very rare, scaly creature found in Asia and sub-Saharan Africa. Pangolins are considered one of the planet's most trafficked mammals. The critically endangered animals have been intensely hunted for their meat and scales, with many of them being traded in Chinese food markets which are often referred to as wet markets because... Working with Greenpeace's investigations unit, Unearthed, we discovered that even after a global ban, pangolins were still being traded. To this day, there is still a debate around the origins of Covid and its traces back to the wet markets of Wuhan in China.[8]

The pangolin investigation was a success and landed a front page story on the i newspaper, subsequently catapulting me into the world of Covid-based investigations. During the same period I met Peter Geoghegan, a fantastic investigative journalist whose work has seen him nominated for British Journalism Awards and the prestigious Paul Foot Award. At the time Peter led Open Democracy's successful 'Dark Money Investigations' portfolio and over the next six months we started to investigate the huge public-sector contracts being awarded by central government as it cast aside normal procurement procedures in a desperate rush to purchase PPE, testing supplies and consultancy support. Billions of pounds of taxpayers' money were spent almost with impunity as Boris Johnson's government struggled to cope with the consequences of the first wave of the pandemic.

Week after week in summer 2020 and through autumn, a familiar pattern was emerging – the DHSC was starting to publish details of huge public-sector contracts being awarded without the normal competitive tendering rules. These contracts were often valued in excess of £100 million and awarded to people with links back to one particular political party – the Tories.

Take, for example, Steve Dechan. Prior to the pandemic he ran a small, loss-making firm distributing medical devices. In May 2020 Mr Dechan's company P14 Medical Ltd was awarded a £156 million contract by the DHSC to supply medical gowns manufactured in China. In previous weeks he had already secured another eye-watering contract from the same government department – a £120 million deal to supply face shields. Dechan was also a Conservative Party councillor and eventual donor to, unsurprisingly, the Conservative and Unionist Party. Off the back of the lucrative PPE deals, Dechan purchased a £1.5 million stately home set within 100 acres of land in the Cotswold countryside. Not bad for the boss of a company that was, pre-pandemic, losing money.[9][10]

In June 2020, Meller Designs, a firm that at the time was selling beauty products, was awarded two contracts by the DHSC with a contract value totalling £81.8 million. These deals were to supply hand sanitiser and face masks. The same company also received a £65.8 million contract to supply face masks in the preceding month. In total, by June 2020 Meller Designs – a beauty products firm – had picked up contracts valued at £148 million to supply PPE to the British government. All of the contracts were awarded without formal competition. The owner of the company was David Meller. Meller was and still is a regular donor to the Conservative Party. At the time of writing this book he had contributed £66,013 into the Tories' coffers. Meller also personally donated to Michael Gove MP and supported his unsuccessful bid to become leader of the Conservative Party in 2016. The relationship between Meller and Gove was rekindled prior to the PPE contract awards and played a pivotal part of Meller Designs' route to riches off the back of the very lucrative PPE contracts, a subject explored in Chapter 2.[11][12]

It wasn't just prospective PPE suppliers that jumped on the government's pandemic gravy train. Medacs Healthcare plc, a healthcare company ultimately controlled by leading Tory donor and former party chairman Lord Ashcroft, received a £350 million contract as part of the government's Covid testing and vaccination rollout. At the time Medacs was a subsidiary of Impellam Group, a FTSE-listed firm whose largest shareholder was Lord Ashcroft, the Belize-based Conservative peer who has donated millions to the party, including more than £175,000 in the year leading up to the contract award. Medacs was criticised in 2019 when a Care Quality Commission report on a homecare service run by the firm was rated "inadequate".

The regulator found "that the care people received was not safe. The majority of people's care calls were not delivered at the time they were expected and people gave examples of where this had impacted significantly upon them and the safety of the care that they received." This scathing report did not stop the DHSC handing them a £350 million contract just months later.[13]

Public anger towards the government was building over its handling of procurement during the first wave of the pandemic. The vast majority of the general public had by now spent months making huge personal sacrifices under difficult emotional and financial circumstances and day after day scandalous examples of huge chunks of the DHSC budget being carved up and distributed to companies with links back to the ruling party were being revealed. At the time Labour MP Rachel Reeves, the then shadow Cabinet minister and now Chancellor of the Exchequer, told me, "People are understandably furious seeing businesses owned and run by the friends and donors of the Tory Party being awarded huge multi-million-pound public contracts throughout this pandemic."[14]

Serious questions remained unanswered. How was this happening? Surely it couldn't be a coincidence? How can one find out what's really going on inside the DHSC and the Cabinet Office?

In October 2020 further clues to help answer these fundamental questions started to be uncovered. Good Law Project, a not-for-profit campaign group based in London and headed up by Jolyon Maugham KC (and whom I would later go on to work for) were embroiled in a judicial review with the DHSC over some of its questionable PPE contracts – they had been leaked a cache of documents from within the heart of government. Good Law Project for the first time revealed details of a special pathway, a secretive procurement channel that designated certain suppliers as 'VIPs'. The leaked files also stated in bold text "high profile contacts require a rapid response", and another document requested civil servants provide the so-called VIPs with an "expedited response".[15]

The leak disclosed on Good Law Project's website and subsequently shared with the *Daily Mail* seemed to me like just the tip of the iceberg. I felt there was likely more to shine a light on. And now here I sit, typing away on this manuscript after what became a four-year-long investigation that unearthed not one, but two controversial 'VIP lanes' and countless examples of cronyism that had roots deep within the heart of government. This book tells not just my story but also recounts the numerous scandals that defined the last half-decade of the Conservative Party's reign.

Chapter 1

The VIP lane

Corruption is a powerful word. A word that evokes images of overseas oligarchs or shady deals taking place between questionable officials in authoritarian countries. Corruption is a complicated word for a journalist and editors, one not to be deployed lightly for obvious reasons. It is a serious accusation and one that will generally draw the eye of an expensive lawyer keen to shut down any suggestions their client may be corrupt. Instead, in this country, we tend to dress up the issue with more woolly words like "old boys' network" or "chumocracy".

Back in 2021, while attending the COP26 summit in Glasgow, the then prime minister Boris Johnson was challenged during a press conference over the numerous scandals connected to cronyism and vested interests that had engulfed his tenure as PM, many of which are covered in this book. Johnson hit back at the suggestions claiming that in his opinion "the UK is not remotely a corrupt country". To believe Mr Johnson's word on this would be a mistake.[1]

One useful benchmark to compare alongside Boris Johnson's assertions is the Corruption Perceptions Index (CPI) published annually by Transparency International, the NGO widely seen as the UK's leading independent anti-corruption organisation. Each year they produce an index that measures how corrupt each country around the world is based on a collection of indicators. The CPI draws its data from 13 different surveys and assessments to generate a score and a rank. Data is gathered on major issues such as the "diversion of public funds", "officials using their public office for private gain without facing consequences" and "whether or not the government has the ability to contain corruption in the public sector".[2]

The United Kingdom's position on Transparency International's corruption index has steadily dropped over the past few years. In 2017 the UK sat joint eighth in the CPI, sandwiched between Germany and the Netherlands. By 2023 the UK had dropped to 20th – its lowest-ever ranking.[3] This accelerated decline has coincided with a number of political scandals. Notably, according to Transparency International, a "stream of revelations about questionable procurement practices during the Covid-19 pandemic."[3][4]

These "questionable" procurement practices referred to by Transparency International predominantly focus on the awarding of government contracts since March 2020 by the DHSC for PPE including face masks, goggles, gloves, gowns, aprons and other medical equipment vitally important in helping to protect NHS staff and the public from catching or spreading the virus.

In April 2020, while the government procurement drive was ratcheting up, the NGO Spotlight on Corruption, whose role includes undertaking meticulous investigation into how the UK manages corruption risks, warned that the method in which government was awarding high-value contracts to companies with conflicting interests could "create substantial problems down the line". The council of Europe and the International Monetary Fund (IMF) also flagged similar concerns during this period. On its current trajectory, the UK was leaving itself extremely exposed to the risk of corruption and cronyism.[5]

The scramble by authorities to purchase critical supplies saw an exponential explosion in the UK's annual spend on PPE products. Budgets leaped from £146 million in 2019 to £15 billion in the reporting period between 2020 and 2021.[5] Granted, this unprecedented increase in spending allowed for much needed supplies for the NHS to be purchased at a time of national emergency; however, it also created an opportunity. With the right political connections within the ruling Conservative Party a small number of individuals were able to syphon off huge chunks of the vast PPE budget and land a once-in-a-lifetime payday. The grotesque profiteering generated from government PPE contracts created scandal after scandal and corruption became an unavoidable subject of discussion inside the corridors of Westminster.[6]

In February 2024 an opinion poll conducted by Savanti and commissioned by the publication Left Foot Forward found that 47% of people questioned thought the current government was more corrupt than previous ones. Only 7% of participants considered the current Conservative Party government less corrupt than its predecessor.[7]

For four years now, I've been investigating the secretive PPE deals – this chapter aims to shed new light and provide useful insight on the government's response to Covid, but, before one gets into the details of these questionable contracts, one must first be reminded of the shambolic state the government's existing stockpile of PPE was in pre-March 2020 – a perilous situation that laid the foundation for the disaster that was to follow.

Pre-pandemic PPE stockpile

In November 2020, eight months after the first lockdown, the National Audit Office (NAO) published its findings on the government pandemic preparations. The conclusions were damning. Prior to the pandemic, the government's structure for stockpiling large quantities of PPE in advance of any potential pandemic was located across two individual programmes. First, the Pandemic Influenza Preparedness Programme (PIPP), which was established to house 760 million items of PPE, and second, the smaller 'EU exit stockpile' – a back-up supply of equipment held in preparation should the UK exit the European Union under a 'no-deal' scenario. Responsibility at this point for managing the purchasing, storage and subsequent distribution of PPE was split across a range of private sector companies and public sector bodies.[8]

PPE for daily use was generally purchased directly by NHS trusts or via a company called Supply Chain Coordination Ltd (SCCL) established by the DHSC to manage the NHS supply chain. In 2019, NHS trusts spent £146m on PPE via these routes.

Overall responsibility for managing the PIPP stockpile sat with Public Health England (PHE) working on behalf of the DHSC. PHE then subcontracted the management to SCCL, which then further subcontracted the responsibility of storing, distributing and managing the day-to-day PPE stockpile to a private company called Movianto. It was both a confusing and complex structure. The DHSC held overall responsibility for the smaller 'no-deal' PPE stockpile.

In theory, the PIPP management established two mechanisms for accessing adequate levels of PPE in the event of an emergency. Firstly, they held supplies in the stockpile managed by Movianto and stored in their vast warehouse, and secondly there was a reliance on 'just in time' contract mechanisms that would enable officials to purchase additional PPE when needed should the stockpile run low.

On 25 January 2020, the then health secretary Matt Hancock sent a WhatsApp message to advisors, which he then posted on his social media feeds. The message was succinct: the UK was ready to withstand "Wuhan coronavirus". The message read: "We are continuing to monitor the Wuhan Coronavirus closely and are taking all necessary steps to protect the public. We have completed 31 precautionary tests and there are no confirmed cases in the UK, the NHS remains well prepared and well equipped to deal with all eventualities".[9]

Hancock's message of reassurance was badly judged. Through February and March 2020, it quickly became apparent the current stockpile of PPE wasn't going to be suitable or resilient enough to withstand demand. The distribution networks established to deliver PPE from the PIPP stockpile promptly collapsed under the sustained pressure.

Pre-pandemic officials had provided an estimate of the quantity of PPE required to be retained in the PIPP stockpile in the event of an outbreak, but under scrutiny it was established that the level of PPE was always woefully short. The PIPP stockpile should have contained 760 million items of PPE, but the NAO discovered that only 401 million items of PPE were held there when the pandemic struck in January 2020 – a shortfall of 359 million items of vital equipment.

For example, according to pre-pandemic estimates the stockpile should have contained 160.6 million aprons, but only 104 million were in stock and available for front-line use. Around 19.3 million gowns should have been available for immediate use from the PIPP stockpile, but it had none – not a single gown to distribute to NHS staff – a vital piece of protective clothing completely missing at a time of national emergency. The PIPP also had a 274-million-item shortfall in the number of gloves required in its own cache, though a further 245 million single gloves were available from the EU exit stockpile if needed.

The lack of gowns available to NHS staff was a significant problem, Internal NHS reports obtained from NHS England and dated 28 March 2020 confirmed the supply chain had "run out of stock on gowns". The DHSC had estimated that the NHS needed to be supplied with 400,000 gowns a day to cope with demand. The shortfall of gowns left NHS staff dangerously exposed. Dr Roberts, an intensive care doctor working in the Midlands, had to take drastic action. She was, at the time, spending 13 hours a day caring for critically ill patients and resorted to making her own out of plastic bin bags. Harrowing images soon circulated around social media of Dr Roberts and her colleagues wrapping pink refuse bags over their heads.[10]

Dr Robert's predicament wasn't an isolated one. The British Medical Association (BMA) conducted a survey of 16,343 doctors in England on 28–29 April 2020 and discovered 48% of all doctors who participated in the survey had resorted to purchasing their own PPE or had relied on donations from charities. In response to the BMA's survey, its then chair, Dr Chaand Nagpaul, said this demonstrated "a damning indictment of the government's abject failure to make sure healthcare workers across the country are being supplied with the life-saving kit".[11]

The Royal College of Physicians surveyed 2,129 hospital doctors in April 2020 and drew a similar conclusion to the BMA – the availability of PPE was having a significantly negative impact on them. More than a quarter – 27% – of doctors could not obtain the correct PPE needed to safely care for patients.[12]

The existing PIPP stockpiles failed to make provision for dentists and pharmacists, who would need PPE to function safely during the outbreak. Furthermore, the PIPP guidelines were drawn up on the basis of the 'reasonable worst-case scenario' in an influenza pandemic and not a coronavirus pandemic – which would require an increased volume of PPE supplies.

DHSC's failure to ensure the country had an adequate volume of PPE supplies in the pre-pandemic stockpile was further compounded when it was discovered that the PPE it did hold was plagued with problems caused by a catalogue of quality and safety issues.

On 21 September 2020 the Government Internal Audit Agency (GIAA) published a report commissioned by the DHSC which examined the "policy decisions, procurement, storage and quality testing" of every PPE item that was previously held in the PIPP stockpile. Its findings were damning. FFP3 face masks, a type of respirator that offers high levels of protection, had elapsed expiry dates and were not replaced and instead the manufacturer just extended the use-by date by "significant margins" and re-deployed them back to NHS staff before being subsequently recalled.

Furthermore, the GIAA discovered the PIPP had retained a stock of "disintegrating" IIR masks, a type of surgical face mask that was previously withdrawn from circulation after they began to fall apart during use.

The GIAA could not find any evidence of "quality testing" on the gloves, safety glasses and aprons held in the stockpile and there was evidence the PIPP's eye protectors were "not appropriate for use in the Covid-19 pandemic", effectively rendering them useless. It was a truly shambolic state of affairs.[13]

Distribution of the stockpiled PPE supplies to NHS trusts at the start of the pandemic was contracted out to, you'll recall, a logistics company called Movianto. Movianto is a former subsidiary of the US private healthcare company Owens & Minor (which subsequently sold the firm in June 2020 mid-pandemic). From the outset, Movianto's ability to respond at the pace required to ensure PPE was distributed in a timely manner to hospitals facing a chronic shortage of supplies was besieged with problems.

Delivery drivers recalled how they often found themselves queuing outside Movianto's Merseyside-based warehouse for hours and hours waiting for PPE to be loaded into their vans, creating an avoidable delay in distribution. At times Movianto staff would load the delivery vehicles with the wrong supplies, creating further logistical headaches.

Ian Rawson, one of the delivery drivers left frustrated by Movianto's strategy, told the *Guardian*, "Nobody knew what they were doing. If this was so urgent to get out, why did they not send more people to get the stuff ready for us?"

Asif Hussain was another driver unimpressed with Movianto's performance. The ex-policeman recalled how "Vans weren't loaded, so you'd wait around for several hours for the vans to be loaded and sometimes they'd give you the wrong equipment to deliver to the hospitals".[14]

Undercover footage obtained by ITV news a few months prior to the pandemic provided a glimpse of the chaos inside Movianto's vast warehouse, where 50,000 pallets of PPE filled row after row of the company's huge racking system. When the shelves became full the PPE was then stored on the ground. PPE spilled into the aisles between the racking system – this would have been a problematic situation as the pallets may have blocked access for forklifts and slowed down the distribution of goods from the warehouse and into the back of the delivery vans patiently waiting outside. ITV's sources said the aisles were blocked for long periods of time, but this is denied by Movianto who said the pallets were only temporarily on the floor as part of a normal inventory checking process (there is no evidence to suggest that they were still there when the pandemic began to unfold). Movianto also said that it complied with its contractual obligations, but in late March 2020 the Army was called in to alleviate the mounting pressure on the crumbling distribution network.[15]

By 23 March 2020 when the first UK nationwide lockdown started, the scandalous lack of PPE reaching the front line was beginning to have devastating impacts on NHS staff. On that same day 62-year-old Dr Peter Tun, an associate specialist in neurorehabilitation at the Royal Berkshire Hospital in Reading, emailed NHS managers pleading for more PPE. The email, published by the *Guardian*, revealed that two colleagues within his department were already self-isolating and his ward had no available surgical masks. Dr Tun warned "if we are not prepared in advance before the ward becomes 'hot' [has confirmed cases], it will be too little and too late". Ten minutes later Dr Tun received a response: his request for additional PPE was denied. According to the trust the masks were "not widely available and need to be used sensibly for those staff most at risk". Two weeks later, Dr Tun tested positive for Covid and ultimately died from the virus on 13 April 2020.[16]

The failure to protect Dr Tun was not an isolated case. On 11 March 2020, NHS Healthcare assistant Thomas Harvey was signed off from duty as he had developed Covid symptoms. According to colleagues who spoke to the BBC, the 57-year-old had been treating a patient who subsequently tested positive for the virus. Shortly after, Harvey also contracted Covid and sadly passed away in early April 2020. Harvey's family believe his death could have been "prevented so easily" if he had been provided with the correct PPE and the right treatment in hospital. Scandalously, the only PPE available to Mr Harvey was a pair of gloves. He had no face mask, face shield or medical gown, leaving him dangerously exposed. In response to Mr Harvey's death, Goodmayes Hospital where he worked claimed they were "following national PPE guidance". All this despite the DHSC claiming they were "working around the clock" to provide the NHS with the equipment they so desperately needed.[6.10] Tragically, throughout 2020, 883 health and social care workers would lose their lives to Covid.[17][18]

In late March and early April 2020 the DHSC finally came to the realisation that the PPE stockpile was not going to be sufficient to meet the demands of the Covid outbreak. Government needed to ramp up PPE procurement to unprecedented levels – the 'Parallel Supply Chain' was established and the infamous VIP lane – or, to give its official name, the "high-priority lane" – was born.

The High Priority Lane

On 1 April 2020, the DHSC announced to the general public the creation of the Parallel Supply Chain (PSC), a new flagship programme that would drastically ramp up the purchasing and supply of PPE. In the weeks leading up to the announcement, DHSC officials, working alongside the consultancy firm McKinsey, had been analysing the likely volume of PPE needed by the government to tackle the pandemic. The global market for PPE had become increasingly more volatile as other countries increased their efforts to secure much needed PPE. It had also been concluded the current stockpiles and the reliance on 'just in time' orders could not possibly keep up with the demand.

The PSC was given five main objectives: plan, source, make, order and deliver. Firstly, using data models generated by the

DHSC and NHS, civil servants needed to plan and prioritise demand for PPE.

Secondly, the DHSC working alongside the Ministry of Defence and Cabinet Office needed to source the vast quantity of PPE needed to meet demand. This was split into three categories: existing supplies managed by the SCCL; suppliers based in China; and new suppliers, which covered companies that offered PPE to the government via its newly established online portal.[19]

Thirdly, the government would encourage existing UK-based manufacturers to repurpose their production lines to make PPE.

Fourthly, the DHSC and SCCL would order, authorise and pay for the PPE.

Fifth and finally, the PPE would be stored, managed and delivered to NHS trusts and Local Resilience Forums.

The PSC was a huge undertaking that required circa 450 staff to manage the process. Civil servants from DHSC were drafted in to help, alongside colleagues from other government departments and private sector consultants. Prime Minister Boris Johnson hired Conservative Party peer Lord Paul Deighton to lead the newly formed PPE programme (Lord Deighton's role is discussed further in Chapter 4).

Official figures report that 37.9 billion items of PPE were procured by the government during the pandemic at a cost to the taxpayer of an eye-watering £12.6 billion.

The government had intended to purchase enough PPE to last four months, but instead in a frenzied market it procured enough volume to last five years. The government's order book included the purchase of 7.5 billion face masks at a cost of £4.2 billion, 14.5 billion gloves at a cost of £1.6 billion, 1.5 billion 'eye protectors' at a cost of £2.5 billion and 700 million gowns at a cost of £2.4billion.[20][21]

Contracts placed with new suppliers via the PSC accounted for 52.4% of the £12.6bn spend whereas contracts with existing suppliers placed by the SCCL accounted for 38.9% and new 'UK make' contracts accounted for the remaining 8.7% expenditure.

In total the DHSC awarded 394 contracts to new suppliers. It had a legal duty to publish the contracts online within one month of making the award. When health officials did eventually start drip-feeding the contracts into the public domain, almost immediately claims of cronyism started flowing.

A pattern quickly began to emerge – companies with no history of supplying PPE to the NHS were suddenly being rewarded with multi-million-pound contracts. Under close inspection the same firms would often have clear links back to the Conservative Party. Suddenly companies with Conservative peers or political donors sitting on their board were being handed astronomical sums of money to supply PPE. The high frequency of contract awards being handed out to politically linked suppliers meant that it was highly unlikely to be a coincidence, but government ministers remained silent. It wasn't until October 2020, when sensitive government documents were leaked to Good Law Project, that we could start to understand the processes that were established to allow potential cronyism to flourish.

Good Law Project obtained a cache of documents that depicted a special pathway: a secretive procurement channel that designated certain suppliers as 'VIPs'. The leaked files also stated in bold text "high-profile contacts require a rapid response". Another document requested civil servants provide the so-called VIPs with an "expedited response".[22]

Pressure from Good Law Project forced the government to admit the existence of a VIP lane (officially named the High Priority Lane) and a month later the NAO published a highly critical investigation into government procurement. For the first time it was now possible to begin the exercise of understanding how and why the VIP lane came to fruition.[23]

In late March 2020, a secretive new procurement route was established. The High Priority Lane was embedded within the Parallel Supply Chain programme headed up by Lord Deighton, on 1 April a dedicated email mailbox was created, and by now a team of civil servants led by Max Cairnduff were seconded into the VIP team to focus entirely on the offers being funnelled into the newly established mailbox.

The VIP lane was created specifically to manage PPE offers that had arrived into the freshly created mailbox via the office of government ministers, MPs, peers and other senior officials. From the outset these offers were considered to be "more credible" simply because of the political recommendations associated with the offer. These bids then became prioritised over the vast majority of PPE suppliers being processed via normal procurement channels who were not aware of the existence of the alternative mailbox and the benefits it could bestow.

Cairnduff arranged for the VIP lane mailbox to be set up on 1 April 2020 and shortly after the 'covid-ppe-priority-appraisals@cabinetoffice.gov.uk' email address was created. Cairnduff shared details of the confidential email address with government ministers and senior officials. Recipients of Cairnduff's 6 April 2020 email included the ministerial offices of Lord Bethell, Michael Gove, Lord Agnew, Jo Churchill and Esther McVey. Cairnduff explained in his email to ministers that "the vast majority" of PPE offers should be directed to the government's public-facing, online portal, before then revealing a priority route for ministerial recommendations. Cairnduff said, "If a PPE offer is a personal recommendation from or contact of a minister or senior official (which if it comes to you

25

it often will be) please direct it to this email address." From the outset companies without the support of a Tory minister were disadvantaged.[24][25]

The VIP lane remained in operation until the end of June 2020. During this time, officials received offers from 493 different suppliers; 208 of these leads came via the offices of ministers, peers or MPs. The government failed to record the source of at least 250 VIP referrals. Ultimately 51 out of the 493 companies succeeded in securing PPE contracts. For every ten companies channelled down the high-priority route one would be awarded a contract from the DHSC.

At first glance, a conversion rate of 1 in 10 or 10% sounds underwhelming – that is, until you compare the results with suppliers trying to bid for PPE through the publicly advertised procurement portal. Here the government received offers from 14,892 companies, but only 104 of these companies succeeded in landing a contract. A conversion rate worse than 1 in 100.[26]

The 51 VIP firms were awarded 115 contracts to supply 7.8 billion items of PPE – the combined contract sum of these deals was a jaw-dropping £3.8 billion.

The DHSC signed off on the multi-billion-pound VIP expenditure over the course of 3 months between late March and late June 2020. During this period civil servants and NHS officials became increasingly frustrated and overwhelmed by the number of politically connected referrals landing on their desk.

Good Law Project for months now had also been raising concerns over the lawfulness of the VIP lane and the potential risk of cronyism surrounding PPE procurement. In spring 2021 its judicial review against the government was going to be heard in the High Court. The public was, for the first time, provided with a glimpse of the inner workings of a procurement system that fast-tracked political connections and at times ignored reputable PPE suppliers.

In November 2020, Good Law Project was granted permission to bring a legal challenge against the secretary of state for health and social care. Earlier in the year the DHSC had awarded highly unusual PPE contracts worth £700m to three companies – Crisp Websites Ltd (trading as Pestfix), Clandeboye Agencies and Ayanda Capital. The contracts awarded to Ayanda and Pestfix were enabled by the High Priority Lane (Chapter 4 discusses the Ayanda deal in more detail).

Good Law Project, led by executive director Jolyon Maugham and legal director Gemma Abbott, argued that the "operation of a secret 'VIP lane', whereby suppliers who had been referred by ministers, MPs and senior officials were afforded more favourable treatment, significantly increasing their prospects of being awarded a contract or contract" was unlawful. The court granted permission and Good Law Project's judicial review was going to be heard at the Royal Courts of Justice in May 2021.[27]

I started working for Good Law Project in November 2020. My role included assisting the legal team in preparation for the upcoming hearing, which I did predominantly by reading through and interrogating the mountains of disclosure provided by the defendants and highlighting any relevant correspondence or evidence that could be of benefit to our legal counsel.

Between December 2020 and May 2021 I, alongside my colleagues, spent countless hours over many days and nights trawling through the thousands of pages of emails, witness statements, spreadsheets, internal reports and text messages disclosed to Good Law Project by the government's legal department.

Thankfully, when the huge cache of documents eventually arrived they were all logged, filed and distributed expertly by Good Law Project's paralegals, ensuring the mammoth task of reviewing the contents wasn't too overwhelming.

For weeks, locked away in my tiny home office, I scrolled through page after page of disclosure, the contents ranging from the mundane to the extraordinary. My colleagues scattered around the country were doing the same, diligently building our argument. I expected to see evidence of ministerial pressure, preferential treatment and examples of problems caused by the VIP lane, but I had underestimated the true scale of the scandal.

On 18 May 2021, the High Court hearing began, enabling certain key government documents covering the PPE procurement period to be shared with the British public.

Multiple examples of civil servants flagging concerns over the VIP lane process were uncovered within days of the High Priority Lane coming into fruition. The sheer volume of referrals from ministers, peers and MPs was hugely problematic. An email exchange between civil servants on 14 April 2020 demonstrated a desperate situation, with officials "drowning in VIP requests". The full exchange reads: "This contact has already been allocated a team member – unfortunately if he jumps to the front of the queue, it then has a knock on effect to the remaining offers of help. We are currently drowning in VIP requests and 'High Priority' contacts that despite all of our work and best efforts do not either hold the correct certification or do not pass due diligence".[28]

Another email exchanged between officials on 29 April 2020 discussing "VIP work" provides an insight into the political leverage being applied. The official claims VIP enquiries "do not always align with priorities in terms of PPE items and volumes but the resultant impact of pressure from ministers can become more of a distraction from the substantive priorities".[29]

By the end of April 2020, civil servants within the PPE procurement cells were being advised to "reduce" the number of cases they assign themselves from companies channelled through "standard" routes to allow more time for VIP cases. The civil servant noted that "VIP cases require about three times the time of a standard case".[30]

Complaints about the VIP lane process were not confined to Whitehall civil servants. NHS officials were also expressing grave concerns. On 20 April 2020, the NHS published its daily Programme Management Update; this report marked "official sensitive" provided a daily update on PPE procurement. The report highlighted a number of risks, including that "VIP escalation is obstructing progress of more viable opportunities for larger/scalable manufacturers" and "VIP escalation is consuming bandwidth for progressing viable opportunities with larger/scalable manufacturers".[31]

I later discovered, courtesy of documents obtained via a Freedom of Information request, that NHS officials flagged the risk of VIPs "obstructing" progress on 12 separate occasions during April 2020.

Good Law Project and its legal team provided evidence to the High Court throughout the May 2021 hearing of the High Priority Lane offering unfair advantage to politically connected VIPs and the evidence disclosed to the public during the hearing was splashed across every national newspaper. A groundswell of pressure was building on the government over its handling of the pandemic – would the High Court agree with Good Law Project's argument? It would take a further eight months before the courts handed down their judgment. In the meantime I turned my focus back to another pressing task.

The VIP Lane Winners

The High Priority Lane closed up shop at the end of June 2020 but by the end of December 2020 the names of the VIP firms who benefited from this process still remained shielded from view. The government stonewalled repeated requests from journalists for the names to be released. By this point the NAO had established that at least 47 firms secured VIP contracts (a figure that would later rise to 51), but the names of the companies and, perhaps more importantly, the names of the politicians who referred them to the VIP mailbox was not public knowledge.

On 18 January 2021, I submitted multiple Freedom of Information (FOI) requests to the DHSC, Cabinet Office and the NAO. I was determined to uncover the missing names and concluded the use of the Freedom of Information Act was the best route to obtaining them. The principles that underpin FOI legislation are simple – "people have a right to know about the activities of public authorities, unless there is a good reason for them not to". The FOI act allows requestors to ask for a myriad of information held by any public authority including copies of emails, text messages, official documents and meeting minutes. [32]

It was clear the DHSC and Cabinet Office had already compiled a list of VIP lane suppliers and that this information was issued to the NAO, which it subsequently used to help inform its November 2020 investigation. My request was simple – I wanted the names of the 47 VIP suppliers.

In theory when a member of the public submits a FOI request to a government department, that department has 20 working days to provide a response, but in the years leading up to the pandemic there was a growing trend for information requests to be refused. Take for example the DHSC – in 2018, only 34% of all FOI requests submitted to the department were "granted in full", by 2019 this number reduced to 33% and in 2020 it dropped further again to 27%.

A refusal from the government wasn't the only risk to consider – in November 2020, openDemocracy discovered the Cabinet Office was operating a secretive unit called the "clearing house" to coordinate and delay the release of potentially sensitive information requested by journalists under the FOI act. Government departments were ordered to share sensitive requests with the Cabinet Office, which would then often block the information from being released.

Shadow cabinet officer Helen Hayes MP said at the time the "blacklisting" of journalists by deliberately interfering with FOI requests was a "grave threat to our values and transparency in our democracy". Journalists working for openDemocracy, the *Guardian*, the *Times* and the BBC found themselves on the receiving end of the clearing house. I later discovered that my FOI requests were routinely submitted to the "Orwellian" clearing house over a five-year period from 2016 to 2021, including "multiple entries" in 2021 while I was trying to obtain the names of the VIP lane benefactors.[33]

Following the January 2021 FOI submission, the DHSC eventually replied three months later on 14 April 2021 and refused my request on the grounds that disclosing the information would "prejudice the commercial interest" of the companies involved. Two weeks later, on 30 April 2021, I appealed the government's decision to refuse my request – they had one month to respond, but ultimately took seven!

On 7 September 2021 the DHSC finally provided a response – it withdrew its previous objection and advised that the names of the VIP lane suppliers would be "published in due course", but stopped short of providing a publication date.

Unsatisfied by the lack of commitment, I again complained to the Information Commissioner's Office (ICO).

On 18 October 2021, the ICO agreed with my arguments and ordered the DHSC to hand over the names – a huge victory for Good Law Project. The ICO, in its decision notice, was highly critical of the DHSC's failure "to comply with its obligations" under the FOI Act and warned the government department that if it didn't comply with its decision it could be found in "contempt of court".[34][35]

On 16 November 2021, the DHSC finally published the names of the companies referred to the VIP lane along with the names of the officials and politicians who provided the crucial referral.[36][37]

The data released by the DHSC was alarming. Initial calculations discovered a staggering £1.6 billion worth of contracts were awarded as a result of referrals from just ten senior Conservative Party politicians. Furthermore, it was only ministers, MPs and peers affiliated with the Tories who were able to refer successful bids – not a single referral from MPs or peers from the Labour Party, Liberal Democrats, Scottish National Party or any other political party succeeded.

In total 15 Conservative Party politicians were named – Dr Julian Lewis MP, Penny Mordaunt MP, Andrew Percy MP, Matt Hancock MP, Steve Brine MP, Esther McVey MP, Grant Shapps MP, Dominic Cummings, Michael Gove MP, Lord Leigh, Lord Feldman, Baroness Mone, Lord Agnew, Lord Leigh and Lord Deighton. [Table 1]

Table 1: Names of suppliers awarded contracts via the High Priority Lane and the source of referral and actual referrer.

Supplier	Source of referral	Actual referrer
Aiya Technology	GCF Covid-19 Enquiries mailbox, Cabinet Office	DHSC PPE Buy Cell
Aventis Solutions Ltd	NHS E&I	Office of Dr Emily Lawson, DHSC
Ayanda Capital Ltd	NHS Shared Business Services	Darren Blackburn, Cabinet Office
Blueleaf Ltd	Keith Lincoln NHS E&I	GCF Covid-19 Enquiries mailbox, Cabinet Office
Brandology Ltd	Dr Julian Lewis MP	Office of Penny Mordaunt MP
Cargo Services Far East Ltd	Andrew Percy MP	Matt Hancock MP
CCS McLays Ltd	Steve Brine MP	DHSC Special Adviser
Community Pharma Co Ltd	Office of Esther McVey MP	Office of Esther McVey MP
Crisp Websites Ltd trading as Pestfix	Office of Steve Oldfield, DHSC	Nick Dawson, NHS E&I
Euthenia Investments Ltd	Office of Lord Agnew	Office of Lord Agnew
Excalibur Healthcare	Matt Hancock MP	Jonathan Marron, DHSC
Eyespace Eyewear	Grant Shapps MP	Not available
GBUK Ltd	Preeya Bailie, NHS E&I	Not available
Global United Trading	Dominic Cummings	Steve Oldfield, DHSC
Headwind Industrial (China) Ltd	Ljupsco Mihailovszki, DIT Budapest	Ljupsco Mihailovszki, DIT Budapest
Hotel Logistics Ltd	Supply Chain Coordination Limited (Responsible for NHS Procurement)	Not available

Ideal Medical Solutions Ltd	Supply Chain Coordination Limited (Responsible for NHS Procurement)	Not available
Invisio Ltd	Supply Chain Coordination Limited (Responsible for NHS Procurement)	PPE Buy Team
JD.COM	Matt Hancock MP	Jonathan Marron, DHSC
KPM Marine Ltd	Office of Dr Emily Lawson, DHSC	Office of Dr Emily Lawson, DHSC
Liaoning Zhongquiao Overseas Exchange Co Ltd	Office of Chancellor of the Duchy of Lancaster	Office of Chancellor of the Duchy of Lancaster
Mazima Markets Ltd	Lord Leigh	Lord Feldman
Mayfair Global	Michael Urwick, Hinduja Foundation	Direct approach
MDS Healthcare Ltd	Referred because the supplier managed a PPE donation made by a third party	Not available
Medicom Healthcare Holding	David Reed, FCDO	GCF Covid-19 Enquiries mailbox, Cabinet Office
Meller Designs Ltd	Office of Chancellor of the Duchy of Lancaster	Office of the government Chief Commercial Officer
MGP Advisory Ltd	GCF Commercial Policy Team	GCF Covid-19 Enquiries mailbox, Cabinet Office
Monarch Acoustics Ltd	Matt Hancock MP	Matt Hancock MP
New Asia Logistic Service PTE Ltd	Dr Andrew Swift	Office of the National Medical Director
Nine United Ltd	Matt Hancock MP	Jonathan Marron, DHSC
NKD International Ltd	Dame Donna Kinnair, RCN	Jonathan Marron, DHSC

The VIP lane

PI4 Medical Ltd trading as Platform I4	Dr Ian Campbell, Innovate UK	Richard James, Cabinet Office
PIF Ltd	Chris Dunn, FCO	Chris Dunn, FCO
Pakan Medical	Christine Emmett, Former HS2 NED	Janette Gibbs, Cabinet Office
PPE Medpro Ltd	Baroness Mone	Office of Lord Agnew
Regal Polythene Ltd trading as Regal Disposables	Chris Hall, Cabinet Office	Chris Hall, Cabinet Office
Rehear Labs Ltd	Supply Chain Coordination Limited (Responsible for NHS Procurement)	Not available
Sanaclis	Supply Chain Coordination Limited (Responsible for NHS Procurement)	Andy Wood, Cabinet Office
SG Recruitment UK Ltd	Lord Chadlington	Lord Feldman
Skinnydip Ltd	Lord Leigh	Lord Feldman
Summit Medical Ltd	Supply Chain Coordination Limited (Responsible for NHS Procurement)	Direct approach
Technicare Ltd trading as Blyth Group Ltd	Office of Gavin Williamson MP	Cabinet Office Correspondence Team
The Paper Drinking Straw Ltd	Stuart Marks	Chris Hall, Cabinet Office
Tower Supplies	Pia Larsen, NHS	Richard James, Cabinet Office
Uniserve Ltd	Lord Agnew	Jonathan Arrowsmith, Cabinet Office
Unispace	GCF Covid-19 Enquiries mailbox, Cabinet Office	GCF Covid-19 Enquiries mailbox, Cabinet Office

Universal Solutions Trading Ltd	HMT Special Advisor	DHSC Special Advisor
Urathon Europe Ltd	Jane Harrison, Supply Chain Coordination Limited (Responsible for NHS Procurement)	DHSC PPE Buying Cell
Visage Ltd	Covid-19 Single Point of Contact mailbox, DHSC	Covid-19 Single Point of Contact mailbox, DHSC
Worldlink Resource	Lord Agnew	Office of Lord Agnew
Wuhan Xiaoyaoyao Pharmaceutical	Office of Lord Deighton	Office of Lord Deighton

In January 2022, two months after the government was forced to publish details of the VIP lane, it was dealt another major blow. The High Court ruled in favour of Good Law Project and declared the VIP lane was "unlawful".

The court found that the operation of a high-priority lane was "in breach of the obligation of equal treatment" and "the illegality is marked by the judgment". The judge also said "there is evidence that opportunities were treated as high priority even where there were no objectively justifiable grounds for expediting the offer" and that officials designated suppliers as VIPs on a "flawed basis".[38]

The combination of the judicial review victory and the publication of the VIP lane winners proved decisive and paved the way for renewed investigations that would ultimately uncover further evidence of cronyism.

PPE Medpro and Baroness Mone

You cannot talk about the VIP lane without discussing the contracts handed to a certain box-fresh company incorporated in London's High Holborn on 12 May 2020 – a fledgling firm that only came into existence six weeks after the first national lockdown. This company, according to the Certificate of Incorporation published on Companies House, had one sole director with significant control of the company – the 44-year-old, Isle of Man-based Anthony Page. The company in question – PPE Medpro Limited.[39]

During the previous week, in early May 2020, the website PPEMedpro.com was registered. An 'off the shelf' website that boasted how PPE Medpro was "a specialist manufacturer of Personal Protection Equipment" went live shortly after. They claimed to be the "go to company for quality and safety" and a large blue rectangle filled the home page declaring to visitors they "can be a hero", before promptly providing a link to view the PPE products up for grabs via the PPE Medpro 2020 catalogue.[40]

The catalogue offered buyers the opportunity to purchase highly desirable PPE products like IIR masks, face shields, goggles, gloves, thermometers, hand sanitiser and, perhaps most notably, much needed gowns. At first glance one could be forgiven if they were initially convinced by the firm's ambitious claims.[41]

PPE Medpro's declaration of being the "go to company" for buyers of PPE was a bold statement and under closer scrutiny turned out to be a complete misrepresentation. PPE Medpro in reality hadn't supplied a single piece of PPE to the NHS or DHSC and certainly had never manufactured any PPE goods at this point.

This however didn't prevent the company hitting the jackpot on 30 May 2020 when, just 18 days after coming into existence, PPE Medpro was awarded an £80.8m contract by the UK government to provide 210 million three-ply medical masks, commonly known as type IIR face masks. The masks were manufactured by Shengyan Medical, based in China's north-eastern Liaoning province and, luckily for PPE Medpro, this deal fell into the category of being 'ex-works', meaning that the UK government were responsible for collecting the masks from the Chinese warehouse and subsequently delivering the goods back to the UK. PPE Medpro in reality was just operating as a middleman – a familiar pattern that would slowly emerge when the PPE contracts procured via the VIP lane were eventually published. In effect, the company didn't actually do anything substantive save for tacking on a profit margin for themselves when, in effect, the government could have procured the masks directly and saved whatever amount PPE Medpro had added to the price.[42]

The rapid rise in fortunes didn't stop there for PPE Medpro as 26 days later, in June 2020, the company was awarded another contract by the DHSC. Again in similar fashion to the previous deal, this was to be handed to PPE Medpro on a plate via a direct award and without a prior call for competitors to bid for the contract. On this occasion the firm was tasked with supplying 25 million sterile surgical gowns at a cost to the taxpayer of exactly £122m.[43]

Miraculously, the company which didn't exist just 44 days previously had amassed lucrative government PPE contracts valued at £203m. The mysterious PPE Medpro was flying high, That is, until 10 weeks later, in September 2020, when one of the most shocking case studies of cronyism in recent British history began to unravel.

During the pandemic, normal procurement procedures were abandoned in favour of direct awards. For the government, this conveniently mitigated the need for the DHSC to publish in advance the details of any potential PPE tenders. The resulting impact often meant that the first opportunity journalists had to report on the latest PPE contracts was to wait for a notice, often referred to as a 'contract award notice' to be published by the Health Department on the UK government's online contracts database. These notices, as previously explained, were often made public many months after the event. This was actually unlawful, but the DHSC became a repeat offender.

On 7 September 2020, the contract award notice detailing PPE Medpro's £122m contract to provide surgical gowns was finally made public and shortly after that Good Law Project, working with Nick Sommerlad the investigations editor at the *Mirror*, quickly established that Anthony Page, the person listed as being in significant control of PPE Medpro, had strong ties to Conservative party peer Baroness Mone and her Isle of Man-based husband Doug Barrowman.[44]

Anthony Page had suspiciously resigned as company secretary of a company called MGM media on 12 May 2020, the exact same day that PPE Medpro was incorporated. MGM Media Ltd is registered at a five-storey, stone townhouse in Edinburgh sandwiched between another equally grand stone building to its right and a KFC to its left. Crucially, MGM was controlled by a certain Baroness Michelle Georgina Mone OBE.

Anthony Page and another of PPE Medpro's directors, Voirrey Coole, both worked in management roles for Doug Barrowman's Knox group – an Isle of Man-based financial services company controlled by Barrowman.

The ties between PPE Medpro's directors – Mone and Barrowman – raised eyebrows, but these links were quickly dismissed. Lawyers representing Mone and Barrowman confidently told the *Mirror* newspaper in early October 2020 that "Baroness Mone has no comment as she has no role or involvement in PPE Medpro. Mr Barrowman is also not involved in the company PPE Medpro and is not a Director or Shareholder."

I, like a lot of people, was not convinced by the rather blunt dismissal by Mone and Barrowman's legal team, but at this point the evidence was not yet available to confidently claim otherwise. The financial and reputational risk posed to journalists from powerful people like Mone and Barrowman willing to use the legal system to bury a story or sue for libel is real, which made gathering more evidence a necessity.

Intrigued by Jolyon Maugham's and Good Law Project's revelations and the robust dismissal from Mone's lawyer, I continued to dig deeper into PPE Medpro as the whiff of cronyism around these deals was potent. Perhaps unsurprisingly, it wasn't long before I had my first breakthrough.

By now it was late November 2020. I was at home working, as usual, behind my desk in my rather cold and often damp office. The phone started to ring and I had to fumble around clearing paperwork off my desk to uncover it. I eventually found it on about the eighth ring and was greeted on the other end of the line by a regular and reliable source. The conversation didn't last long, but they did provide a valuable tip-off. They claimed PPE Medpro secured its £203m PPE contracts courtesy of being referred through the 'VIP' lane.

This was important because, by this point in late 2020, the National Audit Office had already confirmed that 47 companies obtained contracts after being funnelled down the VIP lane or the High Priority Lane as it was also known. Crucially however, only two of the 47 company names had been revealed courtesy of Good Law Project's ongoing legal work – they were Ayanda Capital and Pestfix (more about them in Chapter 5). Had I just discovered that PPE Medpro was a third name to add to the list?

I urgently needed to verify the claims and spent the next fortnight speaking to other sources, trawling online for any further clues, reading through parliamentary questions, NAO reports and anything else that I thought could provide confirmation. Still, nothing came to bear. Out of ideas, I decided to try my luck with the Cabinet Office press team and asked a simple question: "Did PPE Medpro get funnelled down the VIP route? Or recommended by ministers?" A few days later I got a response.

In true Cabinet Office fashion, the response started with the usual waffle and background information; in this instance it was an extract from a Westminster Hall debate and a speech on the VIP lane by Cabinet Office minister Julia Lopez. It began, "In order to manage this influx of offers, a separate mailbox was set up to handle this area of work. This is the oft-cited 'high priority lane", which colleagues on the other side of the House have sought to portray as something far more sinister than it was. Far from being a 'secret referrals lane', this mailbox was in part a triage for directing more credible leads..." and on it went. By now I had become familiar with this type of rebuttal, full of political soundbites but lacking in substance. Just as I was about to dismiss the entire contents of the email, I scrolled to the bottom of the message and the following words leaped out of the screen: "On your question about Medpro. Medpro did go through the high priority inbox". I was amazed they answered the question. The gamble had paid off, and I got the verification I needed to finally publicly reveal the name of another VIP lane beneficiary – PPE Medpro Ltd.

By now, it was early December and I had started freelancing for Good Law Project. I shared my discovery with Jolyon Maugham and we both agreed that we should reach out to David Conn, the *Guardian*'s brilliant senior investigative reporter. It quickly became apparent to David and me that this story wasn't going to be straightforward.

Yet again Baroness Mone, Doug Barrowman and PPE Medpro's legal team came back to the *Guardian* with strong statements distancing Mone and Barrowman from Medpro. Similarly, Medpro tried to distance itself from the VIP lane and government ministers and peers.

Our piece did allow us to reveal for the first time that PPE Medpro's offer to supply PPE was processed through the VIP channel; however, we still had to refrain from stating Mone and Barrowman were involved in the deals because they both continued to blatantly mislead via their lawyers in response to David's questions.

Remarkably, lawyers for Mone and Barrowman told the *Guardian* "that neither of them is an investor, director or shareholder in PPE Medpro, and that neither had any role or function in the company, or in the process by which the contracts were awarded".

PPE Medpro's response was equally misleading. The *Guardian* piece quoted Anthony Page, Medpro's director, claiming "that neither he nor anybody involved with PPE Medpro approached any MPs, peers, government officials, ministers, NHS staff or other health professionals as part of making the approach to the government to supply PPE", and that all discussions were with the "correct and appropriate individuals" within the civil service.

PPE Medpro claimed they were "not awarded the contract because of company or personal connections to the UK government or the Conservative Party".

The DHSC was equally as unhelpful and declined to say why the PPE Medpro bid was given preferential treatment.

The *Guardian* article was finally published on 21 December

2020. While I was pleased with my small role in exposing PPE Medpro's links to the VIP lane, my bigger goal was to unequivocally uncover and disclose the political links between Medpro and the Conservative Party. I wanted to know who referred PPE Medpro to ministers (was it Baroness Mone?) and which ministers then subsequently fast-tracked the firm through the VIP lane. I did eventually find those missing pieces of the puzzle, but it took another *11 months* to do so.[45]

In January 2021, one month after the Guardian piece was published, I submitted a Freedom of Information (FOI) request to the DHSC.

Throughout my career I've consistently utilised the FOI Act to prise important information out of government bodies with a fair bit of success. Despite the obvious limitations and the real threat from government ministers developing new tactics to thwart the release of sensitive or embarrassing documents, it remains one of the best tools available to an investigative journalist and I'm always surprised that more of my fellow journalists do not make use of it. However, if you intend to obtain high public-interest material via FOI, it's now unfortunately commonplace to expect a decent response from the government to take months and possibly years – gone are the days when you could submit your questions and receive an email containing all the documents you request 20 working days later – obtaining the names of the 47 VIP lane firms and the politically connected people who fast-tracked them was no different. It took ten months for the DHSC to provide a request that should have taken one month.

In mid-November 2021, when Good Law Project and I finally got our first glimpse of the companies fast-tracked down the High Priority Lane, the first company I scrolled to on my computer screen was PPE Medpro. While I already had the proof that they'd benefited from the VIP lane, there was a bigger prize I was seeking to confirm: *who* had got the company into the "special inbox"? Courtesy of my slow internet speed and my eager curiosity (after all, I'd waited nearly a year for this moment), what should have taken just a matter of seconds to scroll down the page seemed to take an eternity. But the wait was worth it. Right there in black and white, printed next to the name of 'PPE Medpro Ltd' under a column titled "source of referral" was the name – Baroness Mone.

We now finally had unequivocal proof that Baroness Mone was involved in referring PPE Medpro to government ministers. The DHSC also cited Conservative MP and Cabinet Office minister Lord Agnew as the "actual referrer" meaning, in short, that Mone had introduced PPE Medpro to Lord Agnew.

The government also provided some waffle about the definition of the various types of referrers. They claimed "The 'source of referral' is the individual or team that identified the organisation and the 'actual referrer' is the individual or team who directed the offer to the high priority (VIP) route."[46]

The bombshell disclosure led the news for the next day or two with decent coverage in the BBC, *Daily Mail*, the *Guardian* and more. At this point you'd think that Baroness Mone would have finally come clean and provided an honest account of her involvement with PPE Medpro. You'd have been wrong. She did not and instead, via her lawyers, she doubled down, telling the *Guardian* that she hadn't lied previously, and said: "Having taken the very simple, solitary and brief step of referring PPE Medpro as a potential supplier to the office of Lord Agnew, our client did not do anything further in respect of PPE Medpro".

Remarkably, when the *Guardian* questioned Mone about the failure to include PPE Medpro on her House of Lords declaration of interests, her lawyers responded by claiming she didn't need to declare the referral because "she did not benefit financially and was not connected to PPE Medpro in any capacity". Words that would later come back and haunt the Baroness and her husband Doug Barrowman.[47]

After my initial collaboration with David Conn in 2020, he continued his incredible journey investigating the PPE Medpro contracts. That journey would end up being a three-year investigation that provided unparalleled insight into the connections between the government, Baroness Mone, Doug Barrowman and PPE Medpro. The inspirational reporting landed David the prestigious Paul Foot Award in 2023 and he continues to this day to publish further bombshell revelations about the cronyism at the heart of these deals. What he uncovered was remarkable.

In January 2022, sensitive files associated with the PPE Medpro contracts with the government were leaked to the *Guardian*. The contents were staggering and for the first time revealed details of Baroness Mone and Doug Barrowman playing a central role in the award of the £203m deals to PPE Medpro. Document after document provided evidence of the pair's secretive involvement. The *Guardian* reported that Barrowman and Mone "were kept informed of specific commercial arrangements about PPE Medpro". Mone was caught sending text messages to members of the PPE Medpro supply chain regarding the £122 million contract to supply surgical gowns and furthermore, Doug Barrowman was "personally involved" in setting up the PPE deals.

During the same week in May 2020 when PPE Medpro was incorporated, the firm established a trading relationship with another company called Loudwater Trade and Finance Ltd. The leaked documents revealed that Loudwater would source the PPE from China, leaving PPE Medpro, Mone and

Barrowman to use their contacts within the UK government to secure a buyer for the PPE procured by Loudwater. Within three weeks of Loudwater and PPE Medpro forming their partnership, the DHSC handed Medpro its first contract valued at £80.5 million to supply 210 million IIR face masks. The second contract with DHSC, worth £122 million to supply surgical gowns, followed shortly after.

WhatsApp messages, reportedly between the PPE Medpro supply chain staff and Baroness Mone in June 2020, sent just days before PPE Medpro were awarded the gowns contract, reveal Mone discussing the size of the gowns required. She also provided a running commentary on when the contract was likely to be issued: "we are just about to take off in the jet. The sizes are in the order. We are waiting for the official PO, this should come in today". A quick reminder, dear reader: Baroness Mone and her partner Mr Barrowman were claiming in that *Guardian* piece they were "not connected to PPE Medpro in any capacity" – a scandalous falsehood.[48]

News that Baroness Mone was affiliated to PPE Medpro despite the many legal rebuttals was enough for Labour peer George Foulkes, officially Baron Foulkes of Cumnock, to submit a formal complaint to the House of Lords Commissioner for Standards. Baron Foulkes said at the time, "If Baroness Mone and her husband were involved in the company then it appears to me that she should have registered that as an interest, and she may have breached the rules against lobbying when she referred the company to the government. And with this conduct and her denials in relation to the company, she may have brought the house into disrepute, so I believe the commissioner should investigate."

Foulkes was supported in his efforts by Tory MP Kevin Hollinrake, who added, "The code of conduct is quite clear that peers must not seek to profit from membership of the house, yet the public record shows that Lady Mone made the initial referral through parliamentary channels, and evidence that she pursued and promoted their application, and that there are connections between her, her husband and the company concerned."[49]

Baron Foulkes's letter of complaint worked and in mid-January 2022, 11 days after the Labour peer's intervention, the HoL Commissioner for Standards launched their investigation into Mone's "alleged involvement in procuring contracts for PPE Medpro".[50]

Fast-forward about two months to March 2022 and the first real evidence of Baroness Mone lobbying Tory ministers was catapulted into the public domain. David Conn and the *Guardian* team were again the journalists shining the light. They uncovered clear evidence of Mone lobbying Cabinet ministers and Conservative Party grandees Michael Gove and Lord Theodore Agnew in the days leading up to the PPE Medpro contracts. Remarkably, this was before the firm had even been incorporated with Companies House!

In fact, Mone sent emails to Agnew's personal email accounts on 8 May 2020 – four days before PPE Medpro had officially come into existence. Baroness Mone started the cosy exchange with: "Dear Theodore, I hope this email finds you well. Michael Gove has asked [sic] to urgently contact you. We have managed to source PPE masks through my team in Hong Kong", concluding with "Hope to see you in the House of Lords when we get out of lockdown. Kindest Regards, Michelle". Agnew replied the same day thanking Mone for her "kind offer" before referring the offer onto DHSC's "Priority appraisals mailbox". The subject header in the email was conveniently changed to include the word 'VIP' and civil servants were urged by Agnew's office to "pick up" the offer from Baroness Mone. The following month, PPE Medpro was awarded its first multi-million pound PPE contract – a now iconic example of the politically focused VIP lane in action.[51]

Mone continued to lobby ministers from May 2020 until February 2021. By this point in the pandemic PPE Medpro appears to have switched focus from flogging PPE and pivoted unsuccessfully into trying to convince the British government to purchase lateral flow tests from them. In one comical and frank email exchange with Jacqui Rock, the NHS Test and Trace chief commercial officer and civil servant, Rock wrote: "Baroness Mone is going to Michael Gove and Matt Hancock today as she is incandescent with rage on the way she believes Medpro have been treated in the matter. It would appear that no one has told them that they have failed anything and they are being, in her words, fobbed off with another round of testing which Porton Down are saying they are identifying sites to set up and don't know when it will be done".[52]

Central to Mone's lobbying for both PPE and Covid testing kits was Michael Gove, but at the time of writing this chapter his communications with the Baroness still haven't been disclosed and remain hidden from public view. My attempts over a two-year period to force the Cabinet Office to publish his emails with Mone were thwarted and a similar fate has met other journalists and MPs who are also attempting to get the emails released. Frustratingly, the Cabinet Office, where Michael Gove was a minister at the time, refused my FOI request to release the emails in question because the contents were commercially sensitive. When I challenged them on this decision, they promptly provided another excuse, which the ICO agreed with, despite the watchdog understanding my frustration with the delays and change in tack by the Cabinet Office. The reason for withholding the emails: "PPE Medpro, a company linked to Baroness Mone, is subject of an ongoing potential fraud investigation by the National Crime Agency (NCA)". This scandal had just taken another Hollywood-style plot twist.[53]

On Wednesday 27 April 2022, the NCA raided several properties associated with the PPE Medpro contracts; these included the Isle of Man and London offices where PPE Medpro was registered and the mansion home belonging to Baroness Mone and Doug Barrowman. Over a dozen NCA officers turned up unexpectedly at PPE Medpro's office seizing documents and electronic devices. Gove and Hancock didn't escape the attention of the NCA; both were interviewed by the crime agency in order for the investigators to better understand how the two PPE contracts were awarded to PPE Medpro and to ascertain if any criminality was involved in the process. The investigation is shrouded in secrecy with the NCA providing very little detail to the public and two-and-a-half years into the investigation the matter is still ongoing with no end in sight. [54][55]

Six relatively quiet months passed by, until in December 2022, Baroness Mone, Doug Barrowman and PPE Medpro exploded back into public focus again courtesy of David Conn's dogged investigation and in the process reigniting the debate surrounding the unlawful VIP lane. *The Guardian* had obtained damning new documentation that showed the eye-watering greed involved in the Medpro deals; according to reports, Baroness Mone and her children "secretly received £29m" linked to the profits made from PPE Medpro government contracts. A HSBC investigation that was leaked to the *Guardian* discovered a complex business structure had been set up by Doug Barrowman which allowed the businessman to funnel tens of millions of pounds of profit generated by the PPE Medpro deal through multiple offshore companies, with about £29 million eventually landing in a trust that directly benefited Baroness Mone and her children. The HSBC report bluntly concluded the deals "suggest a UK peer in the House of Lords has benefited from a contract with the UK government". In total, Barrowman made staggering profits of £65m from the PPE contracts before subsequently transferring £45.8 million into his personal bank account, and subsequently then transferring £29 million into the Keristal Trust controlled by Mone in October 2020.[56]

For what seemed like weeks after the *Guardian* published its latest PPE Medpro exposé, Baroness Mone trended across social media platforms, forcing the Baroness in December 2022 to take a leave of absence from the House of Lords. The Tory peer vowed to "clear her name of the allegations that have been unjustly levelled against her".[57]

A few weeks after the latest media storm surrounding PPE Medpro and its benefactors the pressure upon them ramped up again when, on 19 December 2022, the government commenced legal action against PPE Medpro. It alleged that the 25 million gowns PPE Medpro had supplied in return for payments totalling £122 million were unusable in a front-line NHS setting and were currently languishing in shipping containers and costing the taxpayer millions of pounds in additional storage costs. It's unclear why the DHSC decided to choose this moment in the midst of public outrage and immense political pressure to announce it was to take legal action against PPE Medpro, but it was clear the government meant business and wanted a full refund of the £122 million it had invested in the gowns, which it now considered to be not fit for use. The DHSC was not satisfied with stopping at £122 million; it also wanted to be fully compensated for the storage costs and subsequent disposal of the gowns, which had spiralled to over £11 million.

In total therefore the government was to pursue PPE Medpro through the legal system for compensation totalling £133.5 million.

The particulars of the claim submitted on behalf of the secretary of state for health and social care to the High Court of Justice were damning. It revealed that on 23 December 2020, DHSC sent a notice to PPE Medpro rejecting the faulty goods. The rejection notice explained that the gowns had been rejected on the grounds that PPE Medpro had allegedly failed to provide the required certification to establish that the gowns "had been reliably sterilised for medical use" and thus rendering them unusable in the NHS. The DHSC also urged PPE Medpro "to collect the rejected gowns at its own risk and expense, or to request that DHSC dispose of them at PPE Medpro's cost" – PPE Medpro didn't take the government up on the offer and dug in for a lengthy legal battle. The case is ongoing.[58]

PPE Medpro rejected the claims made by the DHSC, stating in its defence that all the gowns supplied to the government "were in accordance with the contract". PPE Medpro went on to say "the said gowns complied in all respects with the contract" and subsequently refuted the allegation that the gowns were not sterile when delivered.[59]

Fast forward to spring 2023, and it was clear Baroness Mone and Doug Barrowman had to take drastic action in order to both improve the public perception of them and also to counter the joint threat of the NCA investigation and the government legal action, but far from coming out publicly to apologise, which could have been a welcomed first step, instead however they resorted to even darker, more sinister and often farcical tactics.

On 19 April 2023, Good Law Project took an unscheduled call on its press phone from a journalist claiming to be making a documentary about the PPE VIP lane. The details were vague, but the journalist claimed that the film might be commissioned by ITV or Netflix. The journalist who called that day was Mark Williams-Thomas and he was keen for an off-the-record chat about the organisation's history of tackling PPE procurement. Throughout my time at Good Law Project it wasn't unusual for journalists to contact us out of the blue, so I agreed to give him a call. Due to diary commitments it would be another month before we eventually spoke over WhatsApp, but in the meantime I conducted some initial background checks on Williams-Thomas.

Mark Williams-Thomas is an interesting character. Born in 1970, he spent 11 years in the Surrey police force; in a career that spanned from 1989 to 2000 he climbed through the ranks to eventually become a detective, but also spent time as a family liaison officer working on child abuse investigations. In 2003 he changed path and launched his television career initially advising on scripts for national broadcasters – nine years later he was presenting his own shows for ITV and BBC, notably a 2012 documentary about Jimmy Saville that landed the former cop multiple Royal Television Society awards. For the next decade Williams-Thomas continued to present TV programmes predominantly for ITV; his back catalogue also included a controversial interview with Oscar Pistorius in 2016, but by 2023 when he first reached out to Good Law Project his TV career was on a downward trajectory.[60]

Old habits die hard for some ex-police officers and Williams-Thomas was no different; while his documentary-making credentials initially checked out, it also became apparent that he owned and ran a private investigation business alongside his business partner Martin Kayes, a cyber security consultant. Williams-Thomas established WT Associates

Ltd in 2007 and the firm trading under the name Specialist Investigations offered a variety of controversial PI services ranging from traditional surveillance, countersurveillance and undercover investigations to more niche offerings of helping clients to manage "critical situations where people have found themselves at the centre of a media storm".[61]

So Mark Williams-Thomas was claiming to be an "investigative journalist" but also a private investigator for corporate clients. This raised a number of alarm bells – which character were we dealing with, the journalist or the PI? I decided to proceed with caution, only discussing what I had already published and placed in the public domain.

On 18 May 2023 I had my first call with William-Thomas and Kayes. The call lasted about 40 minutes and we continued to correspond over WhatsApp and email for about a month after the call – it became apparent that the pair didn't have much insight into the world of PPE procurement, but it wasn't completely clear at this point in time if they were just jumping on the bandwagon in an attempt to launch a TV comeback or if something more sinister was afoot. I do remember feeling uneasy about the initial call; they seemed very keen for a face-to-face meeting and it seemed the PIs already knew that I lived in Yorkshire, despite Good Law Project being London based. This is not something I had disclosed, and although it wouldn't take a mastermind to figure out, the suggestion did unnerve me slightly.

Crucially, in June 2023 Martin Kayes, while driving with Mark Williams-Thomas, sent me a WhatsApp message – they were keen for Good Law Project and me to share any information we had regarding the PPE Medpro's contracts. We declined and distanced ourselves from sharing any information we had on PPE Medpro – my gut feeling was they weren't being honest, and I was right.

In mid-July 2023, PPE Medpro took the unusual step of issuing a press release. The dramatic email claimed "PPE Medpro and its investigative team have spent the last 12 months undertaking a thorough forensic investigation into the role of government departments, the Cabinet Office, ministers and officials involved in PPE Procurement. Later this year, we will release our findings which make for very concerning reading. We believe that our findings may well reveal corruption and criminal activity". PPE Medpro, Mone and Barrowman had launched their comeback and almost instantly after reading the email I had a sneaking suspicion that Williams-Thomas was involved.

The next day I messaged Martin Kayes and asked him how the "Netflix documentary" was coming along and if he had seen the PPE Medpro press release. My message seemed to alarm Kayes, who I think was still trying to remain in the shadows. Within 48 hours of my message they were forced to confess that Baroness Mone and Doug Barrowman were funding their documentary, something they failed to declare when they unsuccessfully tried to prise information about PPE Medpro out of me in the previous months.

Kayes also admitted that Mone and Barrowman had hired Williams-Thomas to investigate a "theft of equipment" from PPE Medpro and to "look into" the cases brought against them by the NCA and the UK government. Laughably, the private investigators still tried to claim the documentary was "independent", although they were concerned with how the commissions from Mone and Barrowman would be "perceived".

I was both furious and concerned. I already had my suspicions around the conduct of Kayes and Williams-Thomas, but I still didn't know what level of corporate spying had occurred. Were they spying on me, Good Law Project or others?

Were they even making a documentary? A few days later I called Martin Kayes, but this time I recorded the call – what Kayes confessed on the call was alarming but entirely in keeping with the underhand tactics deployed by Mone and Barrowman since the outset of the pandemic.

Kayes revealed a pattern of highly unethical operations spanning many months being conducted by Williams-Thomas on behalf of Mone and Barrowman. The "theft" that Kayes claimed Williams-Thomas was investigating wasn't, in fact, a theft. Instead, the ex-detective was being paid by Barrowman to hunt down the suspected source who had been leaking information to the *Guardian* for years. Secondly, Williams-Thomas was hired to guide Mone and Barrowman as they attempted to orchestrate a comeback – he was instrumental in organising the now notorious interview between Mone, Barrowman and the BBC's Laura Kuenssberg which eventually aired on 17 December 2023.

If you watch the interview with Kuenssberg closely you can see Williams-Thomas dressed in a dark coat and backpack lurking in the background as the BBC host greets Mone and Barrowman – conveniently Williams-Thomas released his "independent" documentary on his own YouTube channel the weekend before the BBC interview aired.

There was clearly huge public interest in exposing the insidious tactics used by the private investigators which could have had potentially dangerous consequences for the sources and journalist involved in shining a light on the unacceptable greed and deceit that sat at the heart of the scandal surrounding Baroness Mone, Doug Barrowman and PPE Medpro.

Just before Christmas 2023, David Conn and I published a report cataloguing Williams-Thomas's various roles for PPE Medpro. At the time of writing, Williams-Thomas continues to work for Barrowman and Mone while also trying to maintain that he is an independent investigative journalist. I am of the opinion that if Doug Barrowman is paying your fee, it is impossible for you to be 'independent' when reporting on this subject.[62]

The PPE Medpro case is shocking and the actions of Mone and Barrowman are inexcusable. Somehow though, they remain the only known VIP lane recipients to currently be under criminal investigation by the NCA. While scrutiny from the NCA is welcomed, PPE Medpro are by no means the only firm that leveraged connections to senior members of the Conservative Party during the early days of the pandemic to gain both access to the VIP lane and the unimaginable profits that ensued from landing large PPE deals.

By design, the VIP lane enabled and even fast-tracked Tory-backed firms over its politically unaffiliated rivals with often disastrous results for the taxpayer. Take, for example, the case of Worldlink Resources, Unispace, Meller Designs, SG Recruitment and Luxe Lifestyle, to name but a few.

Worldlink Resources

The Hong Kong-registered Worldlink Resources Limited was awarded two contracts worth a combined value of £258 million from the DHSC to supply PPE during the first wave of the pandemic.

The deals were secured by Worldlink after they were successfully referred to the VIP lane by Conservative peer Lord Agnew; however, this declaration by DHSC of Agnew's referral in response to my FOI request only provides a small glimpse into the events that unfolded prior to Worldlink being fast-tracked into a world of unimaginable wealth.

This story begins with a former dog food seller called Zoe

Ley and the former Conservative Party MP and minister Brooks Newmark. Prior to the pandemic Zoe Ley, a former investment banker from London, ran a successful dog food company called Rockster. The organic food brand sold luxury goods to a host of London's A-listers, who would often leave glowing reviews on Rockster's website. Not content with just selling pet food, however, on 1 May 2020, while the country was still grappling with the first national lockdown, Ley decided to branch out and incorporated a new business, which she named Life Partners Limited, and immediately set about brokering PPE deals with the UK government acting as a "bridge" between the DHSC and Worldlink Resources.[63]

Brokers like Ley were a common feature in PPE deals during the pandemic and if you wanted to increase your chances of being fast-tracked onto the VIP lane, having a political ally would certainly boost your chances. This case was no different, and Zoe Ley partnered up with Brooks Newmark to do just that.

Brooks Newmark was the former Conservative Party MP for the constituency of Braintree. He served as an MP for ten years between 2005 and 2015. He was succeeded by James Cleverly in the 2015 general election. During his time as an MP, he also served as the minister for civil society under the leadership of David Cameron.

Newmark's ministerial career was short lived and in 2014 he stood down after he was caught sending explicit messages to an undercover reporter at the *Mirror*. The following year Newmark also stepped down as an MP.[64]

After leaving office, Newmark established his own consultancy business and registered Brooks Newmark & Co. Ltd in May 2015. Companies House records show Newmark's fledgling business remained dormant throughout 2015–2019, before suddenly trading again in the May 2020 accounting period with just £100 capital. May 2020 was of course the same month Zoe Ley established her PPE brokering business and the duo soon formed an unlikely alliance. It would take another year before Ley and Newmark's lobbying efforts were revealed to the world, all courtesy of dogged reporting by journalist Gabriel Pogrund and his colleagues at the *Sunday Times*. They had obtained key email correspondence between the brokers and a number of senior Conservative ministers which provided valuable insight into Ley and Newmark's lobbying operation.[65]

On 26 May 2020, Brooks Newmark reached out via email to Matt Hancock's special advisor, or SpAd as they are known in Westminster. The email, labelled CONFIDENTIAL, immediately launched into a sales pitch urging the UK government to source PPE from Worldlink Resources. Newmark brags in the email that he had already made Matt Hancock and Michael Gove aware of the deal which could "supply the UK government with PPE in volume and the long term". Newmark claimed that if the UK government placed a contract with Worldlink Resources the Exchequer and ultimately the taxpayer could reap the benefit of "savings of several hundreds of millions of pounds" – a bold statement that ultimately fell woefully short on delivery. Newmark concluded his email by urging the SpAd to discuss his proposal with Matt Hancock, Michael Gove, Liz Truss and Lord Deighton – the Conservative peer hired by Boris Johnson to oversee PPE procurement.

The next morning, an impatient Newmark directly lobbied Matt Hancock about the same deal. The former health secretary responded the same day with a simple response, "Thanks. Definitely one for the PPE team who are firing on all cylinders now". Twenty minutes later, Newmark sent another candid email across to Hancock urging for somebody to "lead the charge in trying to seriously explore this option". Shortly after *that* Hancock obliged, and his SpAd forwarded the request onto Lord Deighton's office with a request for Deighton to look into Newmark's PPE proposal "urgently".

The unrivalled and uninterrupted access available for Newmark and Ley to multiple Tory ministers during a time of national emergency proved decisive – just three days after Hancock's intervention, Worldlink Resources was rewarded with a PPE contract by the DHSC to supply 90 million goggles at a cost of £178 million.[66]

It soon became apparent for the government that the deal brokered by Newmark and Ley was a disaster for the taxpayer. The 90 million goggles provided by Worldlink under the deal had a shelf life of just two years, and when the goggles landed in the UK in bulk it became obvious to officials that the certification provided couldn't demonstrate appropriate evidence that they met strict 'anti-fogging' guidelines – a fundamental requirement that ultimately delayed the PPE from being issued to the NHS.

The DHSC scrambled to conduct additional "acceptance testing" on Worldlink's goggles – a process that only concluded 21 months after the contract was placed and just a matter of a few months before the PPE passed its expiry date.

The DHSC allowed some of the goggles to be distributed to front-line staff. Officials confirmed to me via another FOI request, however, that only 1.3% of the 90 million ordered were dispatched, resulting in potentially 88 million goggles going to waste at a staggering cost to the taxpayer.[67]

Despite the incredible waste, Worldlink Resources was paid the full contract value of £178 million, creating eye-watering profits for Zoe Ley and Brooks Newmark.

Newmark's consultancy business, which was dormant in the

four years before the pandemic, saw a big change of fortune. Capital and reserves at Brooks Newmark & Co. jumped from minus £2,318 to plus £2.3 million in 2021. For Zoe Ley the rewards were even bigger. Her newly incorporated company Life Partners Ltd lodged gross profits of £22.9 million in its first year of trading – for simply brokering deals for medical equipment. The following year, after the PPE bonanza had run its course, the turnover at Ley's company plummeted from £23 million in 2021 to just £47,485 in 2022.[68]

In July 2020, during the same month that the DHSC transferred an initial £59 million to Worldlink Resources, Ley spent £7.25m purchasing an extravagant stately home in Berkshire dubbed "one of the most prestigious rectories in Britain".[69]

At the time of writing, Ley and Newmark appear to have avoided any legal or financial repercussions. Following the problematic contract, Newmark was investigated in November 2023 by the Office of the Registrar of Consultant Lobbyists (ORCL) over his involvement in the Worldlink contract. The watchdog, which published its findings in February 2024, confirmed Newmark's consultancy business received payment from an "overseas company" linked to the contract. Newmark, who was represented by law firm Carter Ruck, disputed claims that he had broken any rules and ultimately, because of a VAT loophole, the ORCL closed the investigation. Dan Neidle of Tax Policy Associates, who first revealed Newmark was under investigation, described the gaps in the lobby rules as entirely legal, but a "serious mistake". He went further and said "this has created a loophole which means that lobbyists acting only for foreign clients don't have to register their lobbying activity. That subverts the purpose of the legislation – the loophole should be closed".[70][71]

As of June 2025, the loophole remained open and lobbyists continue to exploit the gaps afforded to them by a weak lobbying act.

Since March 2020 and the first nationwide lockdown, nine Conservative Party donors, peers or MPs have been investigated by the OCRL including Mohamed Amersi, Mustafa Mohammed, Owen Paterson MP, Samir Jassal, Stephen Brine MP, Lord Andrew Feldman, Baroness Michelle Mone, Brooks Newmark and David Cameron MP. All of the investigations have been linked to lobbying activities related to companies attempting to secure lucrative government Covid-related contracts.

Only one out of ten of these investigations resulted in OCRL taking further action. Owen Paterson MP was issued a penalty notice and fined £7,500 for a breach of the lobbying act following his lobbying of health ministers on behalf of Randox Laboratories Ltd.

This book will explore most of these cases in later chapters.[72]

Meller Designs

David Meller is a British businessman in his 60s who over the past decade has forged close ties to the Conservative Party. Meller has consistently drip-fed cash to the Tories since 2009. Overall, Meller has topped up the party's coffers with donations totalling £63,000.

Notably, Meller became particularly close to one Conservative Party MP – the MP for Surrey Heath, Michael Gove.

Meller has personally donated to Gove on two separate occasions: first, a £1,500 donation in 2009 and second, a £3,250 cash donation in 2016 to help fund Gove's unsuccessful leadership campaign. Meller acted as the finance chair for Gove's bid to succeed David Cameron. Gove eventually lost out to Theresa May.[73]

Meller's other roles include being the trustee of the right-wing think tank The Policy Exchange, which was founded by Gove in 2002. Additionally, in June 2013, Meller accepted the position of non-executive director of the Department for Education's board. Michael Gove was the secretary of state for education at the time.[74]

When the pandemic struck in 2020, Meller and Gove's paths would cross again – the outcome of which would prove to be exceptionally lucrative for David Meller and his company, Meller Designs Ltd.

Meller Designs Limited is a business that's been trading since 1913, specialising in fashion accessories and hosiery. In 2019 the firm reported a respectable turnover of £12.8 million and generated £182,674 gross profit. This followed similar results in both 2017 and 2018 accounting years. 2020 however, was going to be a year like no other for Meller Designs and its owners. The company decided to establish a PPE division and promptly began issuing PPE proposals to government officials in March 2020.[75]

Frustrated by the lack of response from officials, David Meller started to lobby Michael Gove (who was minister at the Cabinet Office during this period), initially complaining that his firm had not received any response from civil servants.

The emails obtained via the *Times* newspaper revealed Meller emailed Gove on 25 March 2020 saying, "This is a really interesting offer, I have not had any responses to my other offers. Only trying to help".[76]

Within hours, the *Times* reported that Meller thanked Gove's office before later emailing to say "look forward to hearing some feedback". Less than two weeks later Meller again resorted to lobbying ministers and on 6 April 2020 he contacted Lord Bethell, a health minister working under Matt Hancock. Also on the call was Lord Feldman – a Tory peer drafted into the DHSC to work as an unpaid advisor. Meller was "looking to deal with a block in ordering" face masks.

The lobbying efforts paid off and at the beginning of May 2020 the DHSC awarded Meller Designs Ltd a £65 million contract to provide 168 million type IIR face masks. A further three PPE contracts valued at £87 million followed in early June 2020. In total, the firm secured PPE contracts from the government totalling £163 million.

In April 2021, Good Law Project was able to reveal that Meller Designs obtained its PPE contracts after being fast-tracked down the VIP lane, but I had to wait until November 2021 and only after a lengthy Freedom of Information battle with the government to find out if any political interference aided Meller's route through it. To nobody's surprise, it had. Meller Designs was "referred" onto the VIP lane by the "office of the Chancellor of the Duchy of Lancaster", the role held by – wait for it – Michael Gove.[77][78]

Following the PPE deals, profits at Meller Designs surged. The firm's annual report, covering the period up to 31 December 2020, saw turnover increase from £12.8m in 2019 to £170m in 2020. Operating profits skyrocketed to £16.4m – an increase of £16.2m compared to the previous year, which equates to a rise of nearly 9000%.

The firm noted in its annual returns that it has supplied "more than 220 million items of PPE to the NHS and other UK health workers, on time and to specification. We are extremely proud of the role we played in the pandemic knowing that NHS workers could go about their vital tasks protected by the equipment we were able to source". This statement, perhaps unsurprisingly, fails to mention two crucial issues. Firstly, PPE valued at £8.46 million supplied by Meller Designs was found to be unsuitable for an NHS setting. Secondly, the DHSC massively overpaid Meller Designs in three out of six of its contracts. Good Law Project investigated the unit prices paid to Meller Designs and discovered that "Of the six contracts, three were paid above the odds, with the contracts awarded at between 1.2 and 2.2 times the average unit price. The average price for medical gowns was £5.87, but the gowns bought from Meller Designs Ltd. cost £12.64".[79][80]

The overpayment to Meller Designs angered the Shadow Chancellor Rachel Reeves, who told the *Guardian* and Good Law Project the "British Public are sick of being ripped off by the Conservatives".

Reeves' solution to this problem would be to appoint a "Covid corruption commissioner", assuming the Labour Party returned to power after the next election. The commissioner would be given the power to interrogate controversial PPE contracts awarded during the pandemic and be tasked with trying to "claw back" some of the excessive profiteering.[81]

Four years on from the PPE contracts, Meller and Gove's relationship continues to make headlines for all the wrong reasons. In February 2024, it was revealed that Michael Gove failed to declare gifts he had received from David Meller in the summer of 2021. While Gove was a minister within the Cabinet Office he accepted hospitality at the West London football club Queens Park Rangers (QPR). The VIP treatment was organised by Jonny Meller, the son of David Meller. David Meller also attended the match with Gove.

According to the code of conduct that all members of Parliament must adhere to, all hospitality received which exceeds £300 in value must be declared in the MPs' register of interests. Gove failed to declare the event, but did subsequently apologise for the "oversight".[82]

Gove's late apology wasn't enough to prevent the Parliamentary Commissioner for Standards launching an inquiry into the apparent breach by the former Cabinet minister. In March 2024, Gove was found guilty of breaching Commons rules by failing to declare the hospitality within 28 days, but no further penalties were imposed on the former minister.

Michael Gove's controversial relationship with VIP lane companies wasn't limited to Meller Designs Ltd. He also played a pivotal role in opening the door for a company called Unispace Global. Unispace would go on to secure the largest PPE VIP lane contracts of any company – worth a staggering £679 million – following the firm's interactions with Gove.

Unispace Global

In November 2022 a luxurious, modern, five-bedroom mansion came on to the market in Dural, a highly desirable suburb of Sydney in the Australian state of New South Wales. The weekend retreat was set within two hectares of land, with huge bifold doors looking out onto the property's private heated swimming pool. The property enjoyed access to its own tennis court as well as a golf driving range. It is a stunning home with a hefty price tag. The day before the property was due to be sold at auction, a mysterious cash buyer stepped in and bought the property for a reported $9.5m, which far eclipsed the asking price. The buyer was Australian businessmen Gareth Hales.[83]

Gareth Hales, alongside his brother Charles, founded Unispace Global, a firm that specialises in interior construction projects for commercial clients. The company operates around the globe, with offices in the US, Australia, Hong Kong and

London. Unispace's clients in the construction industry include numerous global blue-chip firms – Deliveroo, Airbus, Hugo Boss and Just Eat, to name a few.[84]

In the UK, the Hales brothers operated out of an office in central London on the banks of the River Thames in a modest, brick-built office complex that enjoyed views of Tower Bridge. Incorporated in 2011, pre-pandemic Unispace was a successful and profitable business. In the last trading year before Covid swept the globe, the firm recorded £88m in turnover and gross profits of £29m, building upon an already profitable 12 months recorded in the previous year, 2018.

In early 2020, the Hales family, like so many of the individuals discussed in this book, pivoted the business away from the world of construction (albeit temporarily) and into the world of PPE procurement. Despite Unispace having zero previous experience supplying much needed medical supplies to the NHS, they managed to skip ahead of the thousands of other firms offering PPE to the British government and were fast-tracked through the VIP lane process. Between April and June 2020 Unispace was awarded multiple PPE contracts from the DHSC worth a combined value of £679 million – the astronomical sum eclipsed the company's previous turnover and catapulted the Hales brothers into a world of unimaginable wealth – the sort of wealth that allows you to purchase a $9.5m mansion in cash just a few years later.[85]

Looking outside the corporate world, Gareth Hales and his brother Charles are senior members of a little-known, strict Christian sect called the Plymouth Brethren Christian Church (PBCC). The PBCC has a reported 50,000 members living predominantly in tight-knit communities within the UK, Australia, New Zealand, Canada and the USA, but smaller memberships can also be found in communities around Ireland,

Italy, Germany, France and further afield in the Caribbean and Argentina. Research by the investigative platform Open & Candid puts the number of UK Brethren members at approximately 15,000 individuals. The PBCC has at times been described as a "cult" by ex-members who have left or been excommunicated from the group (a term which the Church describes as "wrong and demonstrably untrue"), which operates in a highly restrictive manner.[86][87]

According to Open & Candid: "It is difficult to understand for the wider public & government that over 99% of the brethren community are born into the brethren, they are educated in brethren schools, they do not attend college or university, they are protected from social media and the news, they cannot attend restaurants or watch TV and they can't associate with non-brethren members. Their families are in the brethren, they attend the brethren meeting rooms numerous times a week. When they leave the brethren schools, they work in brethren-owned companies. They shop in brethren run shops. They are groomed to stay in the brethren and are informed that the world outside the brethren, is the world of the devil. Their future wife or husband will need approval of church elders, they will need approval of where they can live and where they can travel. Access to computers & mobile phones will come with strict controls on what they can access".[88]

The claims made by Open & Candid are not all accepted by the PBBC. For example, on the PBCC website the group discuss their role in society and refutes any claims they operate separately from the local community: "We live and work with people of all walks of life in regular neighbourhoods, towns, and cities worldwide. We help our neighbours, and they help us. We actively seek opportunities to contribute to our local communities and to be of service".

When asked about how the PBBC interacts with technology and the internet they said: "We use technology in our personal and professional lives, including mobile phones, laptops, and the internet, similar to the general population. Historically, it is true that we have been cautious in embracing new technologies, always with a view to protecting our families. "However, it'd be pretty tricky to get by in today's day and age without the help of technology".

Since 2002, the PBCC has been under the strict control of one man – Bruce Hales. According to reports, the 71-year-old Australian, who has a taste for private jets, wields "great powers" over the PBCC membership. You will often find a portrait of Bruce Hales, referred to as the "Elect Vessel", hanging in the living room of Brethren member households. Bruce Hales has four sons, including Gareth and Charles Hales, the founders of Unispace Global.[89]

Remarkably, firms owned by Plymouth Brethren members scooped up multiple UK government contracts during the pandemic. In total, deals valued at more than £2 billion to supply PPE and Covid tests were awarded to companies linked to the PBCC. The Hales family had strong ties to many of the successful companies, which included the £679m Unispace deals as well as the huge £947 million contracts to Medco Solutions and the sizeable £272 million contract to Sterilab Services, which was to provide Covid tests for the NHS Test and Trace programme.

Although Brethren ideology is on the political right, members are discouraged from voting in general elections and from donating to political parties, so the PBCC adopt different tactics to wield influence among the ruling Conservative Party.

The PBCC, unlike traditional donors to the Tories, has the benefit of numbers – 15,000 loyal members willing to obediently follow the orders from the Brethren 'elders'. This was put into action during the 2010 general election, when Brethren members took to the streets delivering thousands of leaflets in marginal seats on behalf of Conservative Party candidates.

According to a report in the *Times*, "When David Cameron was coming to power, the Brethren were suddenly told to leaflet as many areas as possible". The message coming from the senior leadership within the sect was clear: "we must help the Conservatives", recalled one ex-member in 2012. Tory MPs accepted high levels of volunteering by means of leaflet drops from PBCC members without having to declare the assistance as a donation with the Electoral Commission.

When in 2012, the PBCC found itself in trouble with the Charity Commission and its charitable status was in jeopardy, multiple Tory MPs, including Peter Bone and Robert Halfon, leaped to the defence of the Brethren – the same MPs who reaped the benefits of the mass leafleting campaign two years previously.[90]

Ten years on from David Cameron's general election campaign, the Hales family still retained access to senior figures within the Conservative Party. On 24 March 2020, one day after the first national lockdown had started and the British public were adjusting to a new, albeit temporary way of life, the Unispace founders reached out directly to Cabinet minister Michael Gove.

The email began, "Dear Mr Gove, Thank you for your time spent with us on the phone earlier. As discussed, our consortium of businesses provides a single source solution for the NHS or Department of Health". Unispace offered Gove the opportunity to buy beds, mobile hand-wash stations, ventilators and, notably, PPE in the form of gloves, hand sanitiser and face masks. The email continued: "Lastly, we have many staff who are ready to work around the clock to provide you all the above and more. All we require is for you [to] give us the nod and put us in touch with the right people to make this happen fast. We can start tonight or tomorrow morning".

The Unispace representative concluded the email in an unorthodox fashion: "We are praying fervently for all men and for you and the Conservative Party at this difficult time. I will be available at any time tonight or tomorrow".

Five days later, at half past midnight on 29 March 2020, Unispace again reached out to Gove. They were frustrated, struggling to "make any headway" with the traditional NHS procurement channel and bluntly asked the minister, "how can we cut through the red tape"? The same day Michael Gove responded, by simply saying "Thank you" and "we will follow up!".

The following morning Michael Gove's office referred the Unispace bid to Matt Hancock's office, who subsequently directed the request to a dedicated Covid email address established by the Cabinet Office. Within 20 days of Gove's team escalating the offer to Hancock's team, Unispace was awarded its first government PPE contract via the VIP lane: a mammoth £239 million award to provide 10 million non-sterile coveralls. Over the course of the next six weeks Unispace continued to regularly pick up new PPE contracts – all awarded without any formal competition.[91]

On 27 April 2020 Unispace landed a £103 million contract to provide face masks. This was promptly followed a fortnight later with a further £104 million deal to provide examination gloves. Three days later, another £9 million contract to supply yet more gloves landed, followed by two additional contracts in early June 2020 totalling £208 million to provide additional gloves (again). By the time government officials had concluded their procurement spree in the later part of 2020, Unispace had been paid £679m, making them the largest recipient by value of VIP lane PPE contracts and inevitably huge profits soon followed.

In December 2020, with the agreement of the DHSC, Unispace Global novated all of its PPE-related contracts to another business controlled by Gareth and Charles Hales – Sante Global LLP. The first annual reports published on Companies House on behalf of Sante Global, which had only been incorporated in May 2020, made for interesting reading. Sante Global recorded £731m in turnover and gross profits of £84m – the profits were shared among the company 'members', of which the Hales brothers are both controlling members.

The DHSC is partly to blame for the excessive profiteering by Unispace. Analysis by Good Law Project found that the contracts issued between April and June 2020 were placed using some of the highest unit prices seen during the pandemic. Good Law Project estimated that the government agreed two contracts with Unispace to provide gloves and gowns at 5.1 and 4.1 times above the average price paid during the same period to other suppliers.

Incredibly, in February 2022, nearly two years after the PPE deals should have been concluded, government health minister Edward Argar had to admit in response to a question from Labour MP Nick Smith that despite the government paying Unispace in full, the firm had only "partially met its contractual obligations". Despite being paid £603 million, Argar said, the NHS had received PPE worth only £484 million. The minister did not explain what had happened to the missing £119 million but did say his department was "working with the company on a commercial resolution for the remainder of the contract". In January 2025, in response to a freedom of information request, health officials confirmed that 11,878 pallets of PPE supplied by Unispace during the pandemic were not used and ultimately destroyed.[92][93]

I think it's fair to say the Cabinet Office really didn't want the emails between Michael Gove and Unispace to see the light of day. For six months they stonewalled my Freedom of Information request, only relenting when the ICO intervened in December 2023. When Good Law Project and the *Guardian* published the emails, the Cabinet Office maintained the position that "ministers had no involvement in these procurement decisions".

On 19 March 2024, the Australian Tax Office (ATO), conducted a surprising and unannounced raid on the Plymouth Brethren's global headquarters in Sydney. According to reports, officers from the ATO were "searching for evidence of misuse of funds by wealthy, high-net-worth Brethren members". The investigators are understood to have seized mobile phones, laptops and other documents from various Brethren-owned locations. At the time of writing, the Australian authorities have remained tight lipped about the specifics of the raid and the progress of its investigation into the Christian group that earned millions of pounds courtesy of the UK government during the pandemic.[94]

Lord Andrew Feldman

Michael Gove was linked to the referral of at least three companies fast-tracked through the VIP lane. Lord Agnew was linked to a further four firms. Joining them at the top of the leaderboard of VIP lane "referrers" is another figure central to the Conservative Party: Lord Andrew Feldman. The Conservative party peer was named by officials as the "actual referrer" of three suppliers into the VIP lane. Those companies were SG Recruitment UK Ltd, Skinnydip Ltd and Mazima Markets Ltd.

The three companies secured DHSC contracts valued at over £60 million following Feldman's intervention alongside Conservative party peers Lord Leigh and Lord Chadlington. [95]

Once described by David Cameron as "one of my oldest and best friends", Feldman attended Oxford with the former prime minister and was put into the House of Lords in 2010. He is director of the Conservative Foundation which aims to raise funds to "safeguard the Conservative Party's finances". During the first wave of the pandemic Feldman took the unconventional step of becoming an unpaid advisor in the DHSC, reporting to health minister and Tory peer Lord Bethell. The move was controversial because Feldman prior to his appointment was managing director of PR consultancy Tulchan, a firm that advised a number of healthcare firms.

Feldman started advising the DHSC on 24 March 2020 and the role concluded on 15 May 2020. The DHSC never formally announced that Feldman was working at the heart of government. It would take an investigation by me and Peter Geoghegan for Open Democracy in November 2020 to finally force the government to go on the record. At the time, Tulchan's clients included providers of PPE, providing a clear conflict of interest. Rachel Reeves, the then Shadow Cabinet Office secretary was the first to raise concerns: "The fact they do so time and time again, and with such little transparency raises grave concerns about what looks to be blatant cronyism". Reeves' worries were certainly valid.[96]

A client of Tulchan's during Lord Felman's reign as managing director was Bunzl Healthcare, a multinational firm with an office in London and a steady track record of supplying healthcare products to the NHS. In March 2020, Bunzl had a major problem: just as the DHSC embarked on its multi-billion-pound PPE spending spree the firm had found itself removed from the government's "approved suppliers list". Fortunately for Bunzl, Lord Feldman was embedded within the DHSC at this point and was on hand to help his client. Emails disclosed to Good Law Project during an August 2021 legal case against the government revealed that Feldman not only helped unblock the approval process for his paying client Bunzl, but that he also played an instrumental role in the firm subsequently landing a £22m government PPE contract.

Feldman emailed the Bunzl CEO, Frank van Zaten, on 22 March 2020 to say, "There have been some historic issues which mean you have been removed from the approved suppliers list. I would like to remedy that as soon as possible." That same day Feldman sent another email to Bunzl management, this time copying in Andrew Wood, a senior government official responsible for procurement on behalf of the Cabinet Office: "I have spoken to him [Wood] about Bunzl and the opportunity for you to supply the UK government with equipment. He will be in touch."

A week passed before Lord Feldman again pressed officials with another email. The peer informed Andrew Wood, "We need to move quickly". Feldman's lobbying efforts succeeded and three days later, on 2 April 2020, the DHSC awarded Bunzl with a £22.5 million contract to supply goggles, masks, gowns, visors and hand sanitiser.[97][98]

When Peter Geoghegan and I pressed Bunzl back in November 2020 about its PPE contracts the firm issued us a stern rebuttal, stating "Bunzl did not receive any orders for PPE from the central government procurement process convened by the Cabinet Office during the pandemic", a response that was wildly inaccurate but unfortunately becoming typical of the disinformation and half-truths that both government officials and prospective PPE suppliers were briefing to journalists.[99]

Another typical example of government ministers providing misleading statements during this period was revealed on 17 August 2021, courtesy of a parliamentary question lodged by the deputy leader of the Labour Party, Angela Rayner. The shadow minister asked her opposite number, the secretary of state for health and social care, a decisive question: "whether the £22.6 million contract awarded to Bunzl Healthcare on 3 April 2020 for personal protective equipment during the Covid-19 outbreak was approved through the eight-stage process to assess and approve offers of support to supply personal protection equipment". The "eight-stage" process referred to by Rayner was a vital due-diligence review conducted on PPE offers by civil servants. It involved important tasks such as ensuring suppliers' bids were compliant with government specification and completing crucial financial background checks on potential suppliers, as well as ensuring they were credible. Earlier in the year Michael Gove boldly told members of the House of Commons that "every single procurement decision went through an eight-stage process". A similar claim was also repeated by Cabinet Minister Julia Lopez and health minister Edward Argar. The response to Rayner's question proved Gove's claims were dramatically false. Not only did Bunzl avoid the eight-stage due-diligence process, but so did 71 other suppliers who, between them, were awarded PPE contracts by the government worth a total of £1.5bn. This included 46 out of the 115 contracts awarded via the unlawful VIP lane.[100][101]

The July 2022 report published by the House of Commons Committee of Public Accounts summarised the abysmal due-diligence failures perfectly: "At no point was consideration given to the extent of the profit margin that potential suppliers would be taking on payments for PPE. Neither was consideration of any potential conflicts between individuals making referrals through the VIP lane and the companies they were referring to. We are therefore unsurprised to see the reports of excessive profits and conflicts of interest on PPE contracts". The National Audit Office was equally unimpressed and concluded the DHSC was "not in a position to fully understand the contract management risks it was exposing itself to".[102]

While Lord Feldman was embroiled in the Bunzl lobbying saga, another embarrassing revelation involving the Tory peer and his lobbying firm was bubbling away under the surface. On 18 November 2020 the BBC's Phil Kemp published a report exploring the £28 million contract awarded by the DHSC to a company called Oxford Nanopore Technologies Limited. The deal to supply diagnostic equipment was handed to Oxford Nanopore on 21 April 2020. By this point in the pandemic, Lord Feldman was fully embedded in his unpaid advisory role in the Health department. Twenty days prior to the contract award, Feldman and Matt Hancock held a meeting with Oxford Nanopore to discuss "testing ambition".[103][104]

Lord Feldman's role with the DHSC ended on 15 May 2020 and he continued he work at his consultancy firm Tulchan. Ten days later the firm unveiled a new client – Oxford Nanopore. In August 2020 the firm secured a second Covid testing contract from the DHSC. This one was a £112 million deal that eclipsed the value of its previous contract and was again awarded without any formal competitive tendering process. Annual reports published by Oxford Nanopore on Companies House demonstrate revenue increasing by 119% between 2019 and 2020, bolstered by its ability to sell Covid testing products to governments.[105][106]

It's worth adding at this point that both Bunzl and Oxford Nanopore were not named on any VIP lane list by the government. It would take another year of investigations before Feldman's involvement was unveiled.

In November 2021, following the publication the VIP lane recipients, Lord Feldman was again back under the spotlight; he had been named as the "actual referrer" of three suppliers. Notably, one was a Hampshire-based company called SG Recruitment UK Ltd which picked up two PPE contracts valued at £50 million to supply hand sanitiser and coveralls.

Prior to the pandemic, SG Recruitment UK was a loss-making business with just £367 cash in the bank. Its main business objective was to provide temporary nursing staff to the NHS. It appears to have had no track record of providing PPE to the British government. It did, however, have a Conservative peer in the directors' boardroom at its Jersey-based parent company, Sumner Group Holdings.[107]

Lord Chadlington, whose real name is Peter Selwyn Gummer, is a director and shareholder of Sumner Group Holdings. Chadlington had also donated over £66,000 to the Conservative Party in April 2020. Lord Chadlington reached out to Lord Feldman via text message:[108][109]

Lord Chadlington: "Andrew I work with a company with PPE. D says you are helping. Shall I put you in touch? Peter"

Lord Feldman: "Yes Please. Best use my DHSC email address AndrewFeldman@dhsc.gov.uk. Thanks very much. Andrew."

Following the text exchange, Chadlington passed Feldman's contact details onto SG Recruitment's boss, David Sumner.

Documents obtained by the *Guardian* revealed that Sumner initially called Lord Feldman on 20 April 2020, before following up with an email the next day. The correspondence sent at 5.10am included details of the PPE that SG Recruitment could provide along with a price list. Sumner noted to Feldman that "Lord Chadlington currently sits on the board" of SG's parent company.

Two hours and 20 minutes later Lord Feldman forwarded the details provided by Sumner on to civil servants managing the "Covid PPE priority appraisals mailbox" – the specific email account set up to manage VIP lane suppliers. Feldman noted in his email to civil servants that this was "an interesting offer from David Sumner who was introduced to me by Lord Chadlington".[110]

Once Feldman had propelled David Sumner's proposal onto the VIP lane team, the PPE contracts soon began to flow towards SG Recruitment. Within five days the firm had landed a £24 million contract to provide coveralls, followed by a £26 million contract a month later on 28 May 2020 to provide hand sanitiser. Internal documents from the DHSC suggest SG contracted the manufacture of the hand sanitiser to a Scottish distillery.[111][112]

The contract between SG Recruitment and the DHSC didn't go smoothly. The NGO Spotlight on Corruption discovered that goods supplied by SG Recruitment costing the taxpayer £26.4m were not fit for purpose. Furthermore, analysis by Good Law Project found that the government paid double the average cost for the gowns supplied by SG Recruitment. The DHSC paid the firm £11.95 for each gown, but the average cost during this period paid to other suppliers was on average £5.87 – an overpayment of circa £10m. The government remains in dispute over the unusable PPE but SG Recruitment, which has changed its name twice since the contract award was wound up in December 2023, is now in liquidation, making it increasingly unlikely the DHSC will recoup any of the £26m lost.[113][114][115][116]

Lord Chadlington's conduct was eventually investigated by the House of Lords standards commissioner but he was cleared of any rule breach. Lord Feldman and Tulchan communications were placed under investigation by the ORCL in November 2020, but the watchdog concluded that neither party breached the lobbying act guidelines, which perhaps tells us more about the lobbying act guidelines than anything else.[117][118]

Luxe Lifestyle

By September 2020, it was becoming apparent that the government was losing the battle to control the narrative around PPE procurement. Week after week regular reports of companies with political connections being awarded huge sums of money to supply PPE were being published online and shared on social media. The constant flow of negative news stories and the ever-increasing risk of judicial reviews alarmed the Cabinet Office, who desperately needed to get a grip on the scandal. It was during this period that Cabinet Office officials made the decision to commission the GIAA to conduct a "targeted review" of six suppliers that were awarded contracts via the VIP lane. The review, according to the GIAA, would consider "recent media and legal scrutiny of contracts awarded to companies whose owners are donors to political parties".

A draft copy of Phase 1 of the report was published on 18 September 2020 and included the agency's analysis of the six "high-profile contracts" – awarded to Pest Fix Ltd, Ayanda Capital Limited, Clandeboye Agencies Limited, P14 Medical Limited, Meller Designs Ltd and Luxe Lifestyle Ltd.

Pre-pandemic, Luxe Lifestyle Ltd operated as a small "design" business and was based on the outskirts of Richmond Park in south-west London. Accounts filed by the firm on Companies House revealed they were losing money and that their accounts were in the red at -£9,017. The supplier's accounts were signed off by the firm's owner and company director, Karen Brost – an American-born fashion designer who is married to hedge fund manager Tim Whyte.[119]

Luxe Lifestyle, having no previous experience supplying PPE to the NHS, was awarded a £25.7m PPE contract by the DHSC in April 2020. Luxe were contracted by the Health Department to supply 10 million FFP2 respirators and 1.2 million gowns.[120]

The DHSC published details of the contract in June 2020 and a week later the decision to place the multi-million-pound contract with a tiny, loss-making supplier hit the headlines, first picked up by *Byline Times* and then legacy news outlet inews. The Luxe Lifestyle deal also caught the attention of Green Party MP Caroline Lucas, who on 6 August 2020 wrote a letter to health minister Jo Churchill. Lucas flagged to the minister the "serious concerns about the government's mismanagement of the purchase of PPE" and cited the Luxe Lifestyle deal as a typical example. This resulting pressure and media attention was enough for the Cabinet Office to include Luxe Lifestyle as a company of interest in the GIAA investigation.[121][122]

The GIAA's assessment of the Luxe Lifestyle deal was alarming. The agency noted Luxe's application was "processed through the VIP channel" following a referral "by an MP". The GIAA discovered the supplier also failed to declare any conflicts of interest. Initially, Luxe Lifestyle wanted to be paid the full contract value of £25.7m upfront, but initial credit checks flagged up some concerns. The agency noted "the original payment was reduced from the 100% initially requested by the supplier, to 50%".[123]

Incredibly, the GIAA discovered that the DHSC didn't conduct some of its due-diligence checks on Luxe Lifestyle until after the contract had been signed. The agency noted, "Further due diligence was carried out after the contract had been signed, with an outcome of 'Red', as the company was only established in 2018 and had only filed abbreviated accounts, which gave limited information on the company's financial viability. As a result, it was suggested that management accounts and additional financial assurances be obtained from the Company, however no evidence, at the time of reporting, was provided to confirm this had been done".

The government's £12.8m upfront payment also caught the attention of Luxe Lifestyle's bank who, according to the GIAA report, put the transfer of money on hold and "also notified the Police", although the funds were subsequently released following an investigation.

The DHSC's decision to fast-track the Luxe Lifestyle contract proved disastrous. Data obtained from Spotlight on Corruption discovered that almost 9 million items of PPE valued at £20 million were not cleared for use by the NHS – a depressingly familiar pattern among VIP lane suppliers.[124]

The management of Luxe Lifestyle's finances still remains shrouded in secrecy. The firm's company accounts covering the key period during the pandemic should have been published on 31 January 2022, but three years later they remain overdue. The directors of Luxe Lifestyle have tried unsuccessfully on two occasions to strike off the firm from Companies House – dissolving the company before the latest accounts are published. As of December 2024, Luxe Lifestyle's latest attempt to be wound down was rejected following an objection to the registrar.[125]

A key question surrounding the Luxe Lifestyle saga still remained unanswered – who was the mysterious "MP" who introduced the supplier to government officials? After a lengthy investigation and legal case I supported while working at Good Law Project, we were able to confirm in February 2023 that it was in fact former Conservative Party MP, minister and party chairman Greg Hands.

Emails obtained by Good Law Project reveal that on 7 April 2020 Hands was lobbied on his personal email account by the then chairman of the local Hammersmith Conservative Party, Mark Higton.

Higton was offering ventilators, Covid tests and six types of PPE; most notably, face masks and disposable gowns, on behalf of Luxe Lifestyle. Higton notes in his email that the company was run by a "friend" who had been "working with the People's Republic of China for over a decade and have [sic] a relationship with the President's Office". Three days later Hands forwarded the offer from Higton and Luxe Lifestyles onto officials working in the Joint Action Coordination Team, a collaboration of civil servants from across Whitehall tasked with sourcing PPE from overseas. Luxe was awarded the ill-fated £25.7m contract two months later.

Interestingly, when Mark Higton was initially approached to comment on the findings, he robustly denied any involvement, claiming he had "never solicited Greg Hands in regards to PPE on behalf of others" – a clear falsehood. A spokesperson for Greg Hands didn't support Higton's claims and confirmed the minister had been contacted, but other than forwarding on the email to the relevant officials "had no further role or involvement in the process and was unaware of any outcome". [126][127]

Knowledge of Greg Hands' referral was ever present among

the procurement teams purchasing PPE because multiple DHSC internal documents leaked to Good Law Project repeatedly used the reference "Minster Hands / Luxe Lifestyles" [sic] when referring to the name of the PPE supplier. Even more remarkable, considering his initial denials, Mark Higton was frequently described as the "Main Supplier Contact" representing Luxe Lifestyle on internal DHSC spreadsheets.

Comically, when the government initially published the names of successful PPE suppliers in November 2021, it listed "Minster Hands" [sic] as the winner of a PPE deal. The Tory minister's name was quietly removed but not before being captured by the Wayback Machine, an online archive which copies and stores historical webpages. The capture from 17 November 2021 prominently displays Hands' name alongside Luxe Lifestyle, Meller Designs and PPE Medpro.[128]

Remarkably, as of January 2025, Luxe Lifestyle has still not published its company accounts covering the time period where it secured the PPE deals – nearly five years ago.

VIP lane data – a moving target

Throughout my time investigating the VIP lane I have noticed inconsistencies with the official number of "VIPs" declared in government reporting. For example, a September 2020 Government Internal Audit Agency (GIAA) report stated "450 companies came through the high priority mailbox (VIP lane) of which 45 were awarded contracts". In November 2020, the DHSC informed the NAO that there were in fact 493 companies processed through the VIP lane, with 47 firms eventually winning PPE contracts. In November 2021 the government revised the official numbers again, claiming 50 suppliers were successful before increasing the total number for the fourth time to 51 firms only a few months later.[129][130]

In early 2022 while investigating PPE contracts for Good Law Project, I was contacted by a whistleblower who was embedded in the PPE procurement team during the pandemic. They had become disillusioned and frustrated by the shifting government position and were outraged by the preferential treatment being handed to politically connected companies. The whistleblower provided a cache of internal government documents and correspondence that gave evidence that ministers may have misled Parliament over the true scale of the VIP lane. The whistleblower also provided examples of government officials manipulating VIP lane data following a scathing NAO investigation. The Department of Health and Social Care disputes the position that other companies may have benefited from the VIP Lane.

One such spreadsheet shared by the leak was titled 'Product_VIP_Atamis' and included details of every company that registered an interest in supplying PPE to the UK government throughout 2020. The mammoth spreadsheet contained 40,000 rows of data split into various categories – supplier name, product ID, contract value and all the other usual information you would expect to see. The contents of one particular column, however, leaped out from the screen. Simply titled "VIP?" it was followed by either a "yes" or "no" answer.

Intrigued, I spent the next few days examining the contents of the spreadsheet. The results were jaw-dropping and revealed the identity of 18 other companies considered to be 'VIPs' by health officials. The additional companies between them had secured £984m in PPE contracts. The overall number of fast-tracked firms now stood at 68 – every contract awarded to these firms was done without any formal competitive tendering process.[131][132]

The analysis flagged a number of contracts that raise

84

eyebrows over the government's decision-making, including a £25 million contract awarded in June 2020 to Hong Kong-based oil and gas firm Jason Offshore Equipment. It took the government 18 months to publish the contract, directly contradicting Boris Johnson's claims in Parliament at the time that all PPE contracts were now "on the record".[133][134]

Furthermore a £96 million contract was awarded to Beijing Union Glory Investment Co. Ltd. An investigation by Josh Layton at *Metro* had previously discovered the firm's registered address was a hotel room in Beijing.[135]

The DHSC initially disputed these assertions but on 11 February 2021, three days after the report was published, they quietly updated the official VIP lane records published on the gov.uk website to include one additional supplier – a company called Technicare Ltd, trading as Blyth Group, that was awarded a £1.7 million PPE contract to supply aprons. Blyth Group secured its route down the VIP lane following a referral from the office of Conservative Party MP and former education minister Gavin Williamson MP.[136][137]

In March 2025, The Covid-19 Inquiry completed four weeks of hearings centred on the controversial procurement decisions made by Boris Johnson's government during the pandemic – of particular interest was the use of a VIP lane.

New evidence published by the Inquiry and analysed by the UK Anti-Corruption Coalition (UKACC) now supports the initial claims made by GLP and in fact goes one step further to reveal the names of at least "20 other suppliers who received 48 contracts worth £1 billion" via the VIP route.

Gavid Hayman, executive director of open contracting partnerships and co-chair of the UKACC, told the inquiry that "we are still not sure we have got to the bottom of all those VIP contracts".

He added: "It appears that the evidence to the Inquiry on VIP Lane suppliers from DHSC conflicts with that of the Cabinet Office.

"The Cabinet Office evidence appears to omit 20 other suppliers who received 48 contracts worth £1 billion according to the DHSC evidence. I am not sure who is right but it is bad that we still don't know for sure five years on. Hopefully, My Lady, you will get to the bottom of it."

The contradicting evidence provided by the Cabinet Office and referred to by the UKACC is in the form of a detailed spreadsheet now made public by the inquiry for the first time.

Remarkably, every PPE supplier awarded a contract by the government during the pandemic can then be filtered into VIP or non-VIP categories, revealing the names of potentially 20 new VIP suppliers.

These 20 suppliers went on to secure PPE contracts valued at £1 billion according to a detailed review conducted by UKACC.

But the confusion doesn't end there.

To date, as we've seen, the names of 51 VIP lane suppliers have been made public by the DHSC. However, earlier in the month, the government's former chief commercial officer Gareth Rhys Williams confirmed to the inquiry that yet another company had mistakenly been missed off the list.

That company was Luxe Lifestyle – as we saw above, a previous investigation by the Good Law Project revealed that Luxe were awarded a £25.7 million PPE deal following an intervention by former Conservative Party ministers and chairman Greg Hands.

Rhys Williams said in his witness statement to the inquiry: "A further HPL company, Luxe Lifestyle was identified in May 2024 following a review of evidence in preparation for this Inquiry."

In March 2025, it was reported that HMRC were investigating Luxe Lifestyle, which led to the arrest of the firm's director Karen Brost on "suspicion of fraud by failing to disclose information, conspiracy to cheat the public revenue and fraudulent evasion of income tax". Her husband, Tim Whyte, is suspected of acting as a shadow director and is also being investigated in connection with the same offences.

Lawyers for Karen Brost told Good Law Project: "that she denied the offences in interview, was released without charge and is not subject to bail. Brost's position is that she is innocent of the offences under investigation". Tim Whyte said he was unable to offer any comment until the HMRC investigation had been concluded.

Furthermore, two officials working in the VIP lane during the pandemic claim another politically connected PPE supplier, Bunzl, was also dealt with via the VIP Lane.

As we saw above, Bunzl had long been affiliated with Conservative Peer Lord Feldman, who was also working as an advisor to health ministers during the pandemic.

Speaking to the inquiry in March 2025, Andy Wood, a deputy director and commercial specialist working for the Cabinet Office, said Bunzl was a "significant, credible offer" that was dealt with via the VIP lane after coming "into contact with the government via ministers and senior officials".

Wood's claim was supported by another senior civil servant, Max Cairnduff, who stated during his hearing on 6 March 2025 that Bunzl was a "really good lead" that potentially came into the VIP lane.

Gavin Hayman, of the UKACC said: "I am not sure who is right but it is bad that we still don't know for sure five years on" the true extent of the VIP lane.

He urged the Inquiry to establish the true picture by

"conducting a comprehensive review of the scale of and outcomes from the VIP Lane".

So far, the names of 51 recipients of the VIP lane have been published by the government, but this could be woefully short with potentially a further 22 PPE suppliers missing from the list.[138][139]

So to recap thus far…

The reporting is only as good as the data

The National Audit office's remit is to "scrutinise public spending" on behalf of Parliament with the intention of holding the government to account; it conducts investigations into government departments and examines whether these departments are being responsible with taxpayers' money. On 26 November 2020 it published the findings of its investigation into "government procurement during the Covid-19 pandemic" and concluded, based on evidence provided by the DHSC and the Cabinet Office, that 47 suppliers obtained contracts after being processed through the VIP lane.

There was one major problem with this conclusion – the government may have fed incorrect or incomplete data to the NAO.[140]

Emails shared by the whistleblower suggested that senior officials at the DHSC and the Cabinet Office knew that many more PPE suppliers were treated as "VIPs" than the 47 names that were reported to the NAO.[141]

Four days after the NAO published its initial findings, on 2 December 2020, Gareth Rhys Williams, the government's chief commercial officer, emailed colleagues regarding VIP data saying: "One question we're going to need an answer to is – what £ value of contracts was given to VIP vendors vs [sic] what

£ value of contracts given to non-VIP, (to match with the 47 vs 104 contracts) best Gareth."

Within an hour of Rhys Williams sending his email JJ van der Meer, the director of the DHSC PPE Buy team replied, "I made some checks but believe we don't have a complete list of the VIP suppliers. Max, would your team have this? JJ".

Van Der Meer was referring to Max Cairnduff, a senior procurement director embedded in the VIP Lane team. Cairnduff responded to van der Meer's comments by saying "A list is being put together at the moment – operationally there wasn't a need at the time."

Rhys Williams emailed again shortly after, bluntly urging officials to ensure their findings matched the NAO PPE spend numbers. The following morning van der Meer urged junior colleagues to ensure their VIP assessment "adds up to the numbers reported in the NAO reports"; he also attached a copy of the NAO report for reference, suggesting the plan was to just make the numbers match.

Other emails provided by the whistleblower demonstrate a frustration among junior civil servants concerned with the multiple requests from senior management to manipulate the data to match what was previously submitted to the NAO; some thought the figures supplied to the NAO may have been fabricated.[142]

It's inconceivable that four years after the PPE contracts were awarded questions remain as to how many politically connected suppliers were – or indeed were not – channelled down the VIP lane. In February 2024, Richard Wald KC, counsel to the UK Covid-19 Inquiry, confirmed the Inquiry would be "scrutinising the reasons for, and operation of, the high priority (VIP) lane" – let's hope the inquiry's legal team can get a definitive answer to this conundrum.[143]

How did ministers not foresee the obvious corruption that would ensue when they allowed the creation of a VIP procurement back channel? They created a system that prioritised a supplier's political connection over its ability to supply much needed supplies. Warning flags raised by civil servants "drowning" in VIP requests went unheard. The NHS repeatedly told officials that VIP suppliers were blocking access to more "viable" and "scalable" PPE offers, but ministers didn't heed the warnings. Established PPE suppliers were ignored, in favour of inexperienced, opportunistic, box-fresh companies that benefited Conservative Party peers and generated eye-watering profits for Tory donors, and 45 out of the 115 VIP lane contracts avoided the vital 8-stage, due-diligence process. From the moment it was conceived the PPE VIP lane was an unmitigated disaster for the taxpayer.

At the end of May 2020, when the government launched the flagship Test and Trace programme – which it pledged to support to the tune of £37bn – ministers at this point could have changed path and implement a fairer, rigorous and transparent procurement process. They did not. Instead, they doubled down on past mistakes and set about establishing a *second* VIP lane. A new, even *larger* VIP lane that ultimately would see companies connected to the Tories land lucrative Covid testing contracts worth an eye-watering £5bn.

Chapter 2

Test and Trace

On 27 May 2020, Secretary of State Matt Hancock spoke to the TV cameras in the now usual and depressingly familiar televised press conference. Standing at the lectern, with the Union Jack hanging from a wood-panelled wall behind him, Hancock announced the devastating news that 37,460 people had so far died from Covid-19 in the UK, including 412 people in the previous 24 hours alone.

Today's press statement also included another significant announcement, and stamped on the front of Hancock's lectern were the words 'NHS Test and Trace'. The next day, on 28 May 2020, the government was going to roll out its new flagship testing programme.

Hancock declared to the British public: "As we move to the next stage of our fight against coronavirus, we will be able to replace national lockdowns with individual isolation and, if necessary, local action where there are outbreaks."

"NHS Test and Trace will be vital to stopping the spread of the virus. It is how we will be able to protect our friends and family from infection, and protect our NHS."

"This new system will help us keep this virus under control while carefully and safely lifting the lockdown nationally."[1]

The purpose of the NHS Test and Trace (NHSTT) system was predominately to ramp up the number of people being tested, to trace people who tested positive and alert people who may have come into contact with a Covid-positive member of the public. The government was desperate to avoid another national lockdown and it saw NHSTT as its solution to avoid a repeat.

The PM, Boris Johnson, appointed Conservative Party peer Baroness Dido Harding to lead the government's new flagship programme, which also had the close involvement of health ministers Matt Hancock and Lord Bethell – another Tory peer.

The sums of money involved were astronomical. £37 billion had been budgeted by the government to support NHSTT – although when the dust settled, circa £29.5 billion of the eye-watering sum was actually spent on the programme, which ultimately failed to prevent the country falling into another national lockdown in winter 2020–2021.[2]

NHSTT was overseen by the DHSC, working in collaboration with PHE – later consumed by the newly formed UK Health Security Agency (UKHSA) – and also local authorities in England. Dido Harding's new testing strategy was heavily reliant on the private sector, despite being branded with the NHS logo.

In fact, officials at the NHS were not happy with the decision taken by ministers to use the NHS name and logo for the Test and Trace project. WhatsApp messages between Matt Hancock, Lord Bethell and Baroness Harding that I obtained via FOI request made that perfectly clear.

During the pandemic the trio of senior officials had a WhatsApp group in operation called 'TnT Matt Dido Jim'. On

15 May 2020, two weeks before the official launch, Harding wrote to Hancock and Bethell saying, "FYI I have just had the expected call from NHS England comms team challenging the use of the NHS brand for Test and Trace. I pushed back really strongly and said it was non-negotiable. Just in case it come [sic] to either of you over the weekend. Hope OK! D".

Half an hour later, Hancock arrogantly replied, "No problem. I own the brand so it's not an issue. They know that so they shouldn't be trying it on".[3]

The largest chunk of the NHSTT budget went on testing services and I will therefore be concentrating heavily on those contract awards. According to the NAO, between 28 May 2020 when the programme was established up to March 2021, contracts valued at £7.8 billion were awarded by the DHSC to support the NHSTT Covid testing requirements.[4]

Huge sums of taxpayers' money were being spent on purchasing Covid tests and the associated lab facilities to analyse the millions of tests being used by the British public. Depressingly, and in similar fashion to the PPE VIP lane saga discussed in Chapter 1, a familiar pattern began to emerge – large contracts were being handed out to companies that appeared to have close connections to the Conservative Party.

In June 2021, while working for Good Law Project, I noticed a strange admission on a civil servant's LinkedIn profile. Simon Greaves had worked on 'VIP stakeholder engagement' and held the job title of 'strategy and stakeholder engagement lead' for the Covid-19 testing programme between April and June 2020.

Greaves said this about his role: "I worked as part of the UK Department of Health and Social Care response to the Covid-19 crisis. My role was to lead VIP stakeholder engagement with Life Science Minister Lord James Bethell, working with diagnostic and biopharma industry executives to build a resilient UK diagnostic centre".[5]

Good Law Project also noticed an email sent by civil servant Max Cairnduff, dated 6 April 2020, that was sent to the ministerial offices of Lord Bethell, Michael Gove, Lord Agnew, Jo Churchill and Esther McVey.

In the email Cairnduff, who as we saw played a senior role in managing the PPE VIP lane, said to ministers: "Please direct offers of testing kits to the following address where they will be triaged: covidtestingtriage@dhsc.co.uk. If they come from a minister/private office then please put FASTTRACK at the beginning of the subject line."[6]

In a similar process to the PPE VIP lane discussed in Chapter 1, senior officials at the DHSC had allowed for the establishment of an email back channel, accessible to ministers. Civil servants were specifically drafted in to handle 'VIP' cases. We had now found clear documentation that the government had created a *second* VIP lane for the procurement of Covid-testing goods. We decided, in that moment, to partner with David Conn at the *Guardian* to reveal the news to the wider public.

Good Law Project's boss, Jo Maugham, said in the *Guardian* piece, "there was clear evidence of a VIP route for companies supplying testing kits. There is an email saying 'fast track' for referrals from ministers, and there was someone dealing with VIP stakeholder engagement. The suspicion is there that contracts were given to companies with VIP connections to ministers. We have heard denials before from the government, but the government has a long history of misleading the public".

But remarkably the government dismissed our report and issued a strong rebuttal to the *Guardian*, stating: "These claims are completely false – there was no high priority lane for testing suppliers. All offers of testing went through the same robust assurance checks and there was no separate 'fast track process'".[7]

By now, I had become accustomed to being lied to by PPE suppliers, but when the government started issuing strong rebuttals claiming the results of my initial investigation were "completely false" it was both disconcerting and surprising. It wasn't long before this unnecessary lie and weak position held by the government began to unravel.

A month later, on 15 July 2021, the *Guardian* revealed how the government gave 'VIP treatment' to a Covid testing company because Matt Hancock was deemed "a good friend" of somebody working with the company, according to emails sent by DHSC officials and obtained by the newspaper.

The Animal Health Trust (AHT) had a laboratory based in Newmarket, West Suffolk – inside Hancock's parliamentary constituency. Pre-Covid, the firm's work focused on medical care for horses and, like Hancock, they had close ties to the horse-racing industry.

According to the *Guardian* in an email on 23 April 2020, a civil servant wrote: "AHT came in direct to SofS [secretary of state] office – someone who works with them is a good friend of his and so they entered the system informally that way... They must have fallen through the records gap if we've not got a trace of them – they've definitely been in touch with us and had VIP treatment."

The following morning, a further email was sent by officials regarding the AHT offer: "We definitely need to capture them in the system somehow, so they receive future comms and offers. Owner [sic] is a friend of SofS, lab is in his constituency/area – so he will get direct feedback on our processes!"

The Guardian also revealed how one email between civil servants discussed the existence of "a stakeholder log" in which officials "capture VIP stakeholders relevant to pillar five [building testing capacity]".[8]

In this instance, AHT did not successfully win a contract from the VIP lane. Still, however, the priority treatment handed to the firm simply because they had the backing of Hancock completely contradicted the government's denials made just a month earlier.

The government was still holding the untenable position that our claims were "completely false – there was no high priority lane for testing suppliers. All offers of testing went through the same robust assurance checks and there was no separate 'fast track process'."

In September 2021, The government finally dropped its denial of the existence of a second high-priority lane after Good Law Project uncovered further email evidence of a "VIP route" discussed by civil servants who were in the process of placing a contract with the York-based Abingdon Health. Abingdon had been awarded a £75 million contract by the DHSC in August 2020 to provide lateral flow devices – a contract that became embroiled in a legal challenge brought by Good Law Project, a case which GLP eventually lost.[9][10]

By 24 February 2022, the government finally let slip the true scale of the NHSTT VIP lane, when Neale Hanvey, Alba MP for Kirkcaldy and Cowdenbeath, asked cabinet officer minister Heather Wheeler a short but effective question: "what his [sic] latest estimate is of the (a) number and (b) value of contracts for the supply of PPE and Covid-19 testing equipment to the NHS which were processed through the high priority lane".

The same day the minister replied: "Between May 2020 and March 2021, 50 suppliers had priority referrals for Covid testing support and were awarded 128 contracts with a total value of £6 billion. All contracts awarded, no matter the route, were rigorously evaluated to ensure that the products that were progressed met the required specification. There was no separate high priority lane or process".[11]

In doublespeak worthy of a George Orwell novel, the minister in the same sentence confirmed there was no "priority lane" despite 50 firms receiving billions of pounds in contracts via "priority referrals".

On 2 March 2022, as soon as I noticed the ministerial response to Hanvey's question I submitted a Freedom of Information request to the DHSC for not only the names of the 50 VIP companies, but also the names of the ministers, MPs and peers who had initially referred them onto the fast-track route.

The DHSC passed the request onto the UKHSA to handle and for the remainder of 2022, the department would try every trick in the book to delay providing an answer to my request.

The DHSC stonewalled. They even tried to withhold the information on cost grounds claiming it would be too expensive to provide the names. They delayed and delayed and delayed. Eventually the ICO ordered the UKHSA to hand over the information.

Ludicrously, the UKHSA told the ICO "the number of electronic files that are relevant to identify the data linked to the request is 70,000 files. It estimates that it will take 4 minutes to assess each file, with a total number of hours projected at 4666.7 at a total cost of £116,666.67 which exceeds the cost limit" – the equivalent of one full-time civil servant spending 9 hours a day searching for 518 consecutive days for the relevant information.

The commissioner wasn't impressed with the government's ridiculous estimates and promptly overruled the decision to withhold the information and on 3 November 2022 ordered the UKHSA to disclose the information within 35 calendar days.

The ICO further warned, "Failure to comply may result in the Commissioner making written certification of this fact to the High Court pursuant to section 54 of FOIA may be dealt with as a contempt of court."[12]

On 21 December 2022, the UKHSA finally relented and handed over the names of the VIP firms alongside the names of the senior officials and politicians who referred them into the high-priority route.

The list was staggering; it quickly revealed that introductions from just six Conservative Party politicians led to 'VIPs' being awarded contracts worth an estimated £5 billion.[13]

Every peer named on the list was a Conservative one, every minister or former minister was from the Conservative Party, every MP named was a Tory MP – in a similar fashion to the PPE VIP lane, only referrals from Conservative Party-linked politicians succeeded in winning contracts. There were no successful awards from suppliers referred by politicians from the Labour Party, Liberal Democrats, SNP or any other political party – the Conservative Party had closed ranks.[14]

The data provided by the UKHSA covered the period in which NHSTT was established in May 2020 through to March 2021. The value of all 158 contracts according to the NAO was £7.8 billion and remarkably the 50 VIP contracts received £6 billion worth of those deals: 77% of all Covid testing contracts placed during this period went to VIPs.[15]

The NAO also pointed out that £4.8 billion of the £6 billion handed to the "priority" firms was done so via "direct awards without competition".

The coordinated method adopted by the government when it finally released the VIP lane details to Good Law Project reeked of ministerial involvement. So a day after UKHSA finally responded to my FOI request, on 22 December 2022, I submitted another request back to them for a copy of all email correspondence relating to the handling of my case. It would take another 13 months for the government to finally respond and of course it required yet another intervention from the ICO.

The emails revealed on 30 November 2022, three weeks prior to disclosure, civil servants began to discuss the "proposed media handling". Officials were devising plans to "control the narrative framing the list and demonstrate our commitment to transparency and openness around Covid-19 decision making" – a laughable position when you contrast this line with the government's initial declaration that Good Law Project's claims of a VIP lane were "completely false". The previous day officials also discussed plans to "inform Parliamentarians in advance of names being released".

On 1 December 2022, 20 days prior to publication, civil servants were monitoring the Good Law Project social media feeds regarding the "Priority lane", noting "The Good Law Project have already tweeted about the 10 day deadline, framing it as being VIP referrers helping suppliers to get into the 'priority lane'. The engagement on this thread is currently quite low but we'll keep an eye on it. If it attracts media interest there is a risk this could be damaging to UKHSA's reputation, especially if we then request an appeal to challenge the ICO's ruling".

On 12 December 2022, nine days before the final publication date, an email with the subject title "URGENT submission to Minister Caulfield – VIP suppliers" discusses the plan to publish the details on the government website prior to handing them over to Good Law Project. This, according to officials, would "help influence coverage" and avoid "driving journalists" to read Good Law Project's "content". This was followed up by another "ministerial information note" on 16 December 2020 to the then secretary of state for health Steve Barclay and Minister Caulfield.

On 19 December 2022, two days before disclosure to Good Law Project, Dame Jenny Harries, the CEO of UKHSA, wrote to health minister Lord Bethell, providing him with an advance warning that they would be soon disclosing the names of the VIP suppliers and referrers to Good Law Project and notably that his name would be included in the list. Matt Hancock was also tipped off by civil servants prior to Good Law Project receiving their response – despite resigning from his role 18 months prior to this date and not currently holding a ministerial position.

Finally, after multiple submissions to ministers and many iterations of the FOI response draft by officials, a final schedule was agreed upon and released to Good Law Project on 21 December 2022. A copy of this is in Table 2 below:

Table 2: Covid testing priority supplier names. Source: UKHSA

Supplier	Identified by	Referrer	Goods/service provided
Abbot Rapid Diagnostics Ltd	Third party contacted NHS England (NHSE) employee and Lord Bethell, Minister for Innovation, DHSC	NHSE employee to covidtesting-triage@dhsc.gov.uk	PCR tests, antibody tests, reagents, and laboratory equipment
Accora Ltd	Supplier contacted Lord Lansley	Lord Lansley to Lord Bethell, Minister for Innovation, DHSC	PCR testing
Aptamer Group Ltd	Supplier self-referred to mailbox covid19triage-service@nhsbsa.nhs.uk	Forwarded from covid19triage-service@nhsbsa.nhs.uk to covidtestingpri-oritycontacts@dhsc.gov.uk	LFD tests

Test and Trace

Berkshire and Surrey Pathology Services	Existing DHSC partner	Existing DHSC partner	PCR testing
Bigneat Ltd	Information not held centrally	Information not held centrally	Laboratory equipment
Bio-Rad Laboratories Ltd	Gareth Rhys Williams, government Chief Commercial Officer, Cabinet Office identified supplier	Gareth Rhys Williams notified Emma Stanton, Director of Supplies and Innovation, NHS Test and Trace. Forwarded to covidtestingprioritycontacts@dhsc.gov.uk	PCR consumables
CAS (Contained Air Solutions ltd)	Existing DHSC supplier	Existing DHSC supplier	Laboratory equipment
Charnwood Campus Management Ltd	Supplier contacted Environment Agency official	Environment Agency official to NHS employee and DHSC officials	Building lease
Dante Labs (Immensa)	Supplier self-referred to online portal	Supplier self-referred to online portal	PCR testing and genomic sequencing
Detact Diagnostics Ltd	Supplier contacted BEIS official	No10 official to Emma Stanton, Director of Supplies and Innovation, NHS Test and Trace	New testing technology
Diasorin Ltd	Supplier self-referred to mailbox covidtestingprioritycontacts@dhsc.gov.uk	covidtestingprioritycontacts@dhsc.gov.uk	Antibody tests

DnaNudge Ltd	Imperial College London contacted Shirley Trundle, Programme Director, National Diagnostic Effort Covid-19	Shirley Trundle, Programme Director, National Diagnostic Effort Covid-19 to covidtestingprioritycontacts@dhsc.gov.uk	PCR tests
Ecolog International (UK) Ltd	Genix Healthcare (third party) contacted Office of Matt Hancock, Secretary of State for Health and Social Care	DHSC official to covidtestingprioritycontacts@dhsc.gov.uk	PCR testing
Eurofins Biomnis UK Ltd	Supplier contacted PHE official	PHE official to covidtesting-triage@dhsc.gov.uk	PCR testing
Hologic Ltd	Existing DHSC supplier	Existing DHSC supplier	Reagents, assays and testing consumables
Hotel Logistics Ltd	Supplier contacted Ministry of Defence (MoD) official	MoD official to covidtestingtriage@dhsc.gov.uk	Lateral flow tests
Health Services Laboratories LLP	Existing DHSC supplier	Existing DHSC supplier	PCR testing
Humasis Co Ltd	Department of International Trade (DIT) official identified list of South Korean test manufacturers	List provided by DIT official to Emma Stanton, Director of Supplies and Innovation, NHS Test and Trace	Lateral flow tests

Test and Trace

Innova Medical Group Inc	Tried & Tested (third party) contacted Dominic Cummings, Special Adviser, No 10	William Warr, Special Adviser at No 10 to Emma Stanton, Director of Supplies and Innovation, NHS Test and Trace	Lateral flow tests
IQVIA Technology Services Ltd	Association of British Pharmaceutical Industry contacted NHSE employee and officials at DHSC and the Office of Life Sciences	Association of British Pharmaceutical Industry contacted NHSE employee and officials at DHSC and the Office of Life Sciences	Evaluation and clinical trial support
LGC Ltd	Supplier contacted Prof John Newton, Director of Health Improvement, PHE	Prof John Newton, Director of Health Improvement, PHE, to covidtestingtriage@dhsc.gov.uk	Laboratory equipment and reagents
LumiraDx UK Ltd	Lord (David) Prior, Chair of NHS England (third party) contacted the ministerial Office of Lord Bethell, Minister for Innovation, DHSC	Ministerial Office of Lord Bethell to Shirley Trundle, Programme Director, National Diagnostic Effort Covid-19	Lateral flow tests
Omega Diagnostics Ltd	Supplier self-referred to mailbox covidtestingpriorit ycontacts@dhsc.gov.uk	covidtesting prioritycontacts @dhsc.gov.uk	Lateral flow tests

Optigene Ltd	Cabinet Office official contacted the ministerial office of Lord Bethell, Minister for Innovation, DHSC, and NHS employee	Cabinet Office official contacted the ministerial office of Lord Bethell and NHS employee	LAMP machines and tests
Origin Ltd	Supplier contacted DHSC official	Office of Life Sciences official to covidtesting-triage@dhsc.gov.uk	PCR tests
Pal International Ltd	Existing DHSC supplier	Existing DHSC supplier	Laboratory consumables
Primer Design Ltd	Existing DHSC supplier	Existing DHSC supplier	Reagents
Pro-Lab Diagnostics Ltd	Existing DHSC supplier	Existing DHSC supplier	Laboratory equipment and PCR tests
Qnostics	Existing DHSC supplier	Existing DHSC supplier	Reagents tests
Roche Diagnostics Ltd	Supplier contacted the ministerial Office of Lord Bethell, Minister for Innovation, DHSC Existing DHSC supplier	Ministerial Office of Lord Bethell to Prof John Newton, Director of Health Improvement, PHE, officials from PHE and Office of Life Sciences, and covidtestingpri-oritycontacts@dhsc.gov.uk	Laboratory equipment and consumables, and antibody tests
Sterilab Services	Supplier contacted official at PHE	PHE official to covidtesting prioritycontacts @dhsc.gov.uk	Laboratory equipment and consumables

Test and Trace

SureScreen Diagnostics Ltd	Liam Fox MP contacted Office of Matt Hancock, Secretary of State for Health and Social Care	Office of Matt Hancock to DHSC officials	Lateral flow tests
Tecan	Existing DHSC supplier	Existing DHSC supplier	Laboratory equipment
The Native Antigen Company	Third party contacted Sir Mark Sedwill, the then Cabinet Secretary, who forwarded directly to his office requesting that they pass on to the appropriate officials	Office of Sir Patrick Vallance, UK government Chief Scientific Advisor covid-testingtriage@dhsc.gov.uk	Reagents
Thermo Fisher Scientific Life Holdings Ltd	Existing DHSC supplier	Existing DHSC supplier	Laboratory equipment
Thriva	Supplier self-referred to mailbox covid-testingtriage@dhsc.gov.uk	covidtesting triage@dhsc.gov.uk	Antibody tests
UNA Health	Existing DHSC supplier	Existing DHSC supplier	Antibody tests and lateral flow tests

11 Universities: University College London, University of Birmingham, University of Liverpool, University of Oxford, University of Southampton, University of Warwick, University of York, University of Manchester, King's College London, Newcastle University, Queen Mary University of London	Existing DHSC partnerships	Existing DHSC partnerships	
Waters Ltd	Ministerial Office of Lord Bethell, Minister for Innovation, DHSC contacted supplier	NHS Test and Trace official to covidtestingprioritycontacts@dhsc.gov.uk	Laboratory equipment
Wolf Laboratories Ltd	Supplier self-referred to online portal	Supplier self-referred to online portal	Laboratory equipment

Innova Medical, Dominic Cummings and Rishi Sunak

According to journalist Richard Brooks, reporting for *Private Eye*, "No company in the history of British civil procurement has been paid so much by taxpayers so quickly as Innova Medical Group Inc."

The story of how a company that was only established in

March 2020 by businessmen Charles Huang and his US-based private equity firm Pasca Capital, and which successfully managed to secure government contracts valued at £4 billion to supply lateral flow Covid tests, reads like a thriller.[16]

Innova relied on controversial intermediaries, a close advisor to the PM and the chancellor of the exchequer to pull off its extremely lucrative payday.

The story begins with Charles Huang, a 60-year-old businessman, whose previous endeavours in the UK include the doomed efforts to save British car manufacturer MG Rover in the early 2000s. In March 2020 he established Innova Medical Group based out of Pasadena in the US state of California.[17]

In his earlier years, Huang studied economics at Wuhan University in China and when the Chinese government disclosed that the same city was the epicentre of the pandemic in early 2020 he "sensed an opportunity" and Innova was born. [18]

Innova and Huang were able to secure exclusive access to lateral flow tests from Chinese manufacturer Xiamen Biotime Biotechnology. The deal enabled Innova to sell the tests globally and they soon began shipping millions of them daily – primarily to the UK.[19]

Within months, huge contracts to supply mammoth quantities of lateral flow devices started flowing from the UK government to Innova. The first contract for £103 million was awarded on 17 September 2020 – not bad for a company that didn't exist prior to March 2020.[20]

Remarkably invoices totalling £149 million were paid by the DHSC to Innova Medical within the first month of the parties going into contract, according to data released to me via a FOI request.

However this was soon eclipsed, and by March 2021,

the government had handed a further six further contracts to Innova totalling an astronomical £3 billion.[21]

By June 2021, Innova had become the foundation of the UK government's mass testing programme as Boris Johnson desperately attempted to keep the economy operational after a number of national and regional lockdowns. But there were major questions regarding the accuracy of the Innova tests brewing away behind the scenes not just in the UK but across the Atlantic in the US – where the US Food and Drug Administration (FDA) on 10 June 2021 took the unusual step to issue a nationwide safety warning that ordered US residents to stop using Innova's Covid tests.

The FDA report was scathing. The agency said it had "significant concerns that the performance of the test has not been adequately established, presenting a risk to health. In addition, labelling distributed with certain configurations of the test includes performance claims that did not accurately reflect the performance estimates observed during the clinical studies of the tests. Finally, the test has not been authorised, cleared, or approved by the FDA for commercial distribution or use in the United States, as required by law."

Furthermore the FDA recommended users of the Innova test should "destroy the tests by placing them in the trash".[22]

The risks of failure associated with Innova's device were considered severe enough for the agency to issue a "class I recall" – the most serious type of recall deployed by the FDA. Innova was also issued with a highly critical warning letter on the same day.

The 10 June 2021 letter from the FDA sent to Innova's chief executive officer Daniel Elliot was scathing and contained details of seven violations of US regulations. A major concern for the US officials was a lack of evidence over the performance of the Innova device, which could in their opinion run the risk of providing "false results" – a potentially disastrous consequence for any use.[23]

The FDA noted about the device: "False-negative results may lead to delayed diagnosis or inappropriate treatment of SARS-CoV-2, which may cause patient harm including serious illness and death. False-negative results can also lead to further spread of the SARS-CoV-2 virus, including when presumed negative patients are grouped into cohorts in healthcare, long-term care, and other facilities based on false test results". Officials gave an equally scathing judgement on the risk of false-positive results.[24]

Questions over the reliability of the Innova tests were also flagged in the UK six months prior to the FDA intervention overseas.

Representatives from the DHSC said the Innova test had already gone through the UK's rigorous Porton Down assessment process. A report published on the evaluation carried out at the Porton Down lab in November showed that the accuracy of the Innova test was on average 79% when the test was given by lab scientists, 73% when administered by health workers and 57.5% when people swabbed themselves.

However, the University of Liverpool analysed data from a pilot scheme rolled out in the city of Liverpool by the UK government in December 2020. The pilot scheme involved the testing of 125,000 residents over a one-month period. The researchers discovered that Innova's lateral flow test "missed 60% of infections in people who were self-swabbing", according to reports.[25]

The numerous alarm bells did not deter the UK government's relationship with Innova and just six days after the FDA recall notice the DHSC awarded another contract to the firm – a

£518 million deal to provide yet more Covid tests was approved on 16 June 2021. By the end of 2021 a further two contracts, valued at an additional cost of £537 million, were also signed between the two parties.[26]

In the space of 15 months Innova Medical, a company that had never traded with the UK government, had secured contracts to supply goods valued at circa £4 billion – in the process, making them by far the biggest recipients of government contracts from the Test and Trace programme. But, a huge question remained: how did they do it?

In December 2022, when the UK Health Security Agency (UKHSA) was forced to come clean and provide me with the names of the Covid testing companies that benefited from its VIP lane, the public could finally begin to find out.

In response to my FOI request, the government confirmed that Innova was a beneficiary of the priority route, a place it secured after being identified by Dominic Cummings – Boris Johnson's closest advisor inside No. 10.

The disclosure also revealed that intermediaries working for a company trading as Tried and Tested lobbied Cummings on behalf of Innova. Cummings then subsequently secured their fast track by referring the offer to William Warr, a health advisor inside No 10, and Emma Stanton, the director of supplies and innovation for NHS Test and Trace.[27][28]

Unrelated to the Innova deal, but a fine example of the revolving door in operation between government and private sector health companies, in November 2020, Stanton would subsequently quit NHS Test and Trace and take up a position at Oxford Nanopore. William Warr would also leave No. 10 for vaccine manufacturer BioNTech. In response to Stanton's departure a DHSC spokesperson told journalists, 'The Department's commercial relationship with Nanopore on testing pre-dated Emma Stanton's arrival and contracts with Nanopore and any other suppliers were subject to usual Government approval processes. Furthermore there's no suggestion that William Warr was involved in the awarding of COVID contracts to BioNTech."[29][30]

Off the back of this latest disclosure, I then sent another FOI request to No. 10 requesting a copy of correspondence between Innova's intermediaries at Tried and Tested and Dominic Cummings – after months of typical wrangling, delays and stonewalling with FOI officials, No. 10 eventually sanctioned the release of the redacted emails to me and the timeline of events revealed how easy it was for Innova's bid to gain 'VIP' traction.

On 29 July 2020, Kim Thonger, director of Tried and Tested (more on him later), contacted Dominic Cummings directly via email. He also CCd in his business partner Charles Palmer also copied into the letter were health minister Matt Hancock and transport minister Grant Shapps. The email contained a letter also dated 29 July, which read:

> Dear Dominic,
>
> I note on the front cover of today's Daily Telegraph that "The chief executive of Heathrow Airport has urged the Government to allow passengers to be tested for Covid-19 on arrival in a trial to rescue the summer tourism season.
>
> We have an accurate, cheaper, quicker solution for airports and airlines. We can help the travel industry to fly again safely.
>
> We are in discussion with the Heathrow supplier and procurement teams, about our rapid 15 minute saliva based antigen test, which gives a result without

requiring a machine or a lab. The test is much cheaper and quicker than a PCR test. It has 96% sensitivity, 100% specificity, 98.98% accuracy. Crucially, because it is an antigen test, and targets the virus itself, it will reliably pick up infection earlier than a PCR or an IgM/IgC antibody test.

We can deliver in volume from August 15th. Samples are available immediately for UK lab testing to verify results we already have. We have exclusive UK distribution rights. Our Californian supplier has exclusive global distribution rights, and is the majority controlling shareholder in the test manufacturing company.

The Californian supplier i referred to above, has previously and repeatedly made an offer, via me to [redacted], Covid-19 Testing programme, to build a factory in the UK, at discovery Park in Sandwich, Kent, to manufacture this test, and our antibody test, to supply UK government, and to supply other private sector clients, such as airlines in the UK and abroad. That Offer stands.

I do hope we may now engage with you to urgently discuss all of the above? We have considerable private sector interest in this new antigen test. It is, if I may use the term you will be familiar with, a true game-changer.

Best regards
Kim Thonger & Charles Palmer Co-Founders:
triedandtested.tech"

Remarkably, within one hour of making the offer, Dominic Cummings referred the brokers on to senior officials and No.

10 subsequently fast-tracked the supplier. William Warr then passed Thonger's details over to Emma Stanton, the senior official leading "testing innovations" for the Test and Trace programme.[31][32]

By 3 August Stanton, Thonger and Palmer had organised further calls with health officials and representatives of Innova Medical and the following month the contracts began to steadily flow to Innova.

One could be forgiven if the investigation into Innova ended at this point, especially as the timeline and the characters involved in the contract awards chimed perfectly with the patterns described in the previous chapter; however, in this case there was another political twist to come, but we would have to wait until Dominic Cummings appeared in front of the Covid Inquiry in late October 2023 – some three years after Innova landed its first government contract.

Prior to Cummings being questioned by the Inquiry, he submitted his "statement of evidence" to the inquiry's legal team. The dossier dated 11 October 2023 and spanning 115 pages provided a fascinating and frank insight into the chaos that engulfed the government throughout 2020 and beyond. Tucked away in paragraphs 91 and 92 was an interesting comment about the Treasury, which at the time was controlled by the chancellor of the exchequer and later prime minister, Rishi Sunak.

The statement read: "Whenever No. 10 asked Sunak's team to fast-track things they did – often having to deal with Hancock's lies and attempts to blame them for failures."

"In the autumn Sunak's team supported me with the mass testing team as we tried to overcome horrific Whitehall bureaucracy, secretly buy hundreds of millions of fast tests before other countries realised their value and there was a PPE-like panic, and build manufacturing capacity in the UK and so on."[33]

This statement by Cummings, claiming that he and Sunak "secretly" purchased huge quantities of Covid tests seemed like a significant confession – I was determined to find out more, so I submitted another round of FOI requests, this time to the Cabinet Office, HM Treasury and the UKHSA.

Three months later and both the Cabinet Office and Treasury failed to provide an adequate response. The Cabinet Office refused to reply on cost grounds. The Treasury declined and said it "does not hold any information in relation to the interpretation of the following remarks made by Dominic Cummings".

However in February 2024, the UKHSA did provide me with a breakthrough. Responding to my request to "provide the name of the company that supplied the tests that are discussed in Mr Cumming's statement" they revealed the names of two suppliers. The first was Innova Medical Group Inc, which they described as simply "Innova". The UKHSA in its response also conveniently provided a link to the contract award, which just happened to be the very first contract awarded to the firm in September 2020 – a contract worth an initial sum of £103.6 million. This contract paved the way for billions of pounds worth of further deals that soon followed.

The news was jaw-dropping. When I approached the Treasury, UKHSA and No. 10 with further questions I was completely stonewalled. Instead of answering my questions, the government decided upon issuing a coordinated statement on behalf of an unnamed government spokesperson, which read:

""We have always said there are lessons to be learnt from the pandemic and we are committed to learning from the Covid Inquiry's findings which will play a key role in informing the government's planning and preparations for the future. While the Inquiry is ongoing, it would not be appropriate to comment."

The government was not denying the truth of Cummings' statement or UKHSA's FOI response, but was now using the Covid Inquiry as an excuse to shield itself from further scrutiny. Let's hope the Inquiry sheds further light on this scandal in due course.

Of course, like the majority of the case studies discussed in this book, Innova and its UK brokers made vast fortunes as a direct result of the government contracts.

For example, Charles Palmer and Kim Thonger, the middlemen who contacted Dominic Cummings in July 2020 via their company Disruptive Nanotechnology (trading as Tried and Tested). Companies House records from December 2019 show Disruptive Nanotechnology had only £85 cash in the bank and owed £3,592 in debts.[34]

Following the eye-watering Innova deals, Disruptive Nanotechnology's profits surged in 2020/21 to £20.5m with a further £18m cash in the bank. The firm claims it has multiple clients, across many different sectors, including "vital national infrastructure, oil and energy, education, finance, healthcare, manufacturing, events, sport, retail and media."[35]

However, Palmer and Thonger's £18m was merely spare change when compared to the astronomical profit margins made by Innova and its owner Charles Huang following Dominic Cummings and Rishi Sunak's Office intervening.

In July 2021, the *Los Angeles Times* revealed directors of Innova Medical were splashing the cash around following the UK government deals that Rishi Sunak team and No. 10 helped to facilitate. The paper reported "executives at a Pasadena startup began flying from Burbank to destinations around the world on a pair of newly registered Gulfstream jets, one a G650 decked out in white plush seats, burnished interiors and other luxury finishes".

Furthermore, the paper reported that two Innova bosses purchased "multimillion-dollar" mansions – and when the individuals were asked to provide evidence that they could afford to purchase the property, they simply "handed over a bank statement showing a $128-million deposit into the company's account from the British government".[36]

Charles Huang earned enough money over this period to enable a £50m donation to be made by his philanthropic foundation to his former university – the University of Strathclyde. The purpose of the donation, according to reports, was for the creation of an institute named after a former supervisor of Dr Huang.[37]

Huang would later boast in a 2022 documentary titled *Asian Inspirations* that his business collected $2 billion (£1.6bn) in profit from his lucrative government deals.

Huang and former directors of Innova are currently fighting each other in multiple legal battles primarily over the astronomical fortunes made by Innova courtesy of the British government.

In a series of extraordinary claims and counter-claims, Huang is accused by former associates and directors of "squandering" or offshoring $1bn of those profits, spending lavishly on private aircraft and a luxurious $18m mansion in Los Angeles. The Innova boss is also accused of splashing cash to buy "homes for his mistresses".

Robert Kasprzak is a former Innova exec currently engaged in a legal battle against Huang. Court documents filed in the US accuse Huang of being "a high-end con artist" who squandered or moved for his own use due to "incompetence, power and greed... more than $1bn of... assets generated from UK sales". He is alleged to have lavished some of the proceeds on luxury purchases including private jets for $70m, the $18m luxury home with a swimming pool in LA known as "the CEO house".

Kasprzak also claims Huang was trying to secure a knighthood from the UK government and has commissioned a biopic about himself, titled *Overnight Billionaire*.

Huang responded to my reporting alongside David Conn in the *Guardian* by denying the claims and alleging that Kasprzak and the former Innova chief executive Daniel Elliott "stole" millions from the company. Kasprzak and Elliott deny those allegations.[38]

In June 2024, after the *Guardian* revealed details of Innova's huge windfall, a source contacted me anonymously and provided me with another insight into the world of Charles Huang.

The source provided me with images of the inside Mr Huang's new private jet, decked out with white leather seats and plush wooden joinery as well as his palatial mansion and its ornate atrium, fitted with a grand staircase and marble floors. In one picture Huang was pictured with his new advisor at the foot of the stairwell. A familiar figure, dressed in a blue suit and white shirt – former prime minister Sir Tony Blair.

After further investigation, journalist Peter Geoghegan and I discovered that Blair has become a paid political and business consultant to Pasaca – the investment group controlled by Huang that also owned Innova Medical.

A spokeswoman for Blair said he met and began working with Huang in 2022 and that the former Labour leader had no involvement in Pasaca's Covid testing business or any interactions with the UK government on its behalf.

"Mr Blair's advice has been around geo-political issues and latterly principally around a technology company spun out of the work done at Strathclyde University. Mr Huang has never asked Mr Blair to lobby or approach the UK government in any way about Covid tests," the spokeswoman said.[39]

The UK government built up a huge stockpile of Covid tests and inevitably large numbers of the tests it procured were "unusable" or ended up being disposed of because their expiry dates were elapsing before the tests were deployed for use.

An FOI request I submitted to the UKHSA revealed at least £246.6 million of taxpayers' money was wasted in this way, procuring 126 million "unusable" Covid tests. The request also revealed Innova Medical was one of the suppliers of the unusable tests; however, it stopped short of explaining how many of the 126 million were supplied by the firm.

Unusable tests were also supplied by Abbott Diagnostics, SureScreen Diagnostics, Tanner Pharma UK, Optigene and Medco Solutions – most of whom we will discuss further on in this chapter.[40]

It's not entirely clear at present whether these firms were at fault for providing unusable tests or if the government was responsible for providing incorrect specifications to the six testing suppliers in question.

A controversial route adopted by the UK government to dispose of the unwanted Innova tests whose expiry dates were nearing was to sell them off cheaply by the pallet load at auction houses. The DHSC placed a contract with Ramco UK in April 2022 to provide auction services for unwanted PPE; the firm would later pivot in 2023 to auctioning unwanted Covid tests.[41]

In December 2023, I was searching through the Ramco UK online auction site and was greeted by multiple lots containing pallets full of unused Covid tests. The bulky boxes which numbered 23 per pallet were all stamped with the familiar NHS Test and Trace logo. By my calculations each pallet contained 9016 Covid tests and bidding for an entire pallet started from as low as £5. The government was writing off a huge loss on every pallet that went through the auction site.

I spent some time depressingly scrolling through the auction site trying to establish who was the initial supplier of the tests; eventually I contacted Ramco just before Christmas 2023 and they confirmed it was the Innova tests, manufactured by Xiamen Biotime. The firm subsequently uploaded a photo onto the auction website containing a label with the words "LATERAL FLOW TEST INNOVA COVID19 RAPID ANTIGEN".[42]

The government VIP lane for testing contracts helped to create the conditions that enabled Innova executives to claim enormous profits and enough money to buy private jets and mansions – and all the while the UK government was offloading pallet after pallet of unused Innova tests at auction houses for a song.

Liam Fox MP and SureScreen Diagnostics

On 3 December 2020, the DHSC placed an order with the Derbyshire-based testing firm SureScreen Diagnostics Ltd. The initial contract commissioned the manufacturer to produce Covid tests in the UK. The deal was valued at £6 million – with the option to purchase further tests.[43]

A few weeks later, on Christmas Eve 2020, the government followed up the initial order with a further contract for £5.3 million to supply "consumables" to support the manufacturing of lateral flow devices.[44]

The initial deals paved the way for a huge contract that was to follow on 15 January 2021 when the government handed a £503 million contract to SureScreen to supply 20 million Covid tests – an eye-watering sum of money that was awarded to the firm without any formal competitive tendering process.[45]

When news of the deal between the DHSC and SureScreen

was announced by the government in early February 2021, government ministers lined up to commend the award. Health and social care secretary Matt Hancock heaped praise on the "brilliant work done by SureScreen, and the contribution it will make to our rapid testing programme". He claimed it was "another example of the home-grown talent, ingenuity and industry that exists here in the UK".

Hancock's colleague and fellow health minister Lord Bethell also weighed in; the Tory peer said he was "hugely grateful for the considerable work" being done by British manufacturers such as SureScreen.[46]

Interestingly Hancock didn't mention in his statement to the press the name of the person who introduced him to SureScreen and paved the way for the half-a-billion-pound contract – more on that later in the chapter.

The contracts quickly became incredibly lucrative for the SureScreen and the Campbell family that owned the firm. Records published on Companies House by SureScreen's holding company, SureScreen Holdings Limited, revealed turnover in 2021 jumped to £150 million, from just £7.8 million in 2020. Profits also surged. Gross profits in 2020 were a respectable £3.9 million, but this skyrocketed to £74.2 million in 2021. SureScreen noted in its annual accounts that the increase in profits was "as a result of the award of a new contract".[47]

SureScreen continued to reap the benefits of the DHSC contracts the following year. Accounts published in 2022 showed turnover increasing to £176 million and gross profit of £69.6 million. The directors again contributed the firm's success to the "continuation of contracts that were awarded in the prior year" – SureScreen were selling lateral flow tests to 60 countries; however, the firm's largest contract came via a £503 million lateral flow contract from the DHSC.[48]

By May 2022, shareholders' funds in SureScreen Holdings topped £90 million and £3 million in dividends was also paid out. In the two-year period covering the pandemic the company reported a gross profit margin of £143.8 million.

So the question remains – how did SureScreen get its foot in the door with the UK government? And how did it subsequently land a place on the VIP lane?

The answer to that question begins with the Conservative MP for North Somerset and former trade minister – Sir Liam Fox.

Liam Fox directly emailed health minister Matt Hancock on 22 June 2020. The email, which I obtained via a FOI request, revealed Fox was lobbying Hancock on behalf of SureScreen. The email, which contained the subject header "BRITISH ANTIBODY TESTS", was very direct and began, "Hi Matt, as you probably know, one of the British companies exporting huge numbers of antibody tests is Derbyshire- based Sure screen. They have performed extremely well in internationally conducted trials. I received the following from their main director David Campbell today..."

Fox then relayed a message from SureScreen director David Campbell to Hancock, which read, "As discussed, we have recently had further validation data coming out of Guy's and St Thomas's, and would like to see if we can proceed with government approval in the UK". Campbell ended his message to Fox with a plea to help unblock the approval process and to "ask that the UK government approve our test for use in the UK/NHS. Our test is very accurate and would deliver both a time and cost saving to the NHS".

Fox then concluded his email to Hancock by requesting if it would "be possible to send this on to PHE and ask them to be in touch with the company. As we enter the next phase I don't think the British people would understand or approve of the widespread export of this capability when we will have a huge need at home".[49]

After Fox's appeal to Hancock, approval of a SureScreen test followed a few months later and the highly profitable contracts began to flow not long after.

Fox's rule was crucial to SureScreen's success – a fact confirmed by government officials when they later told me in December 2022 that the referral by the Tory MP for North Somerset played a pivotal role in the firm landing a place on the VIP lane.[50]

SureScreen's contract with the government to supply Covid tests commenced in January 2021 was intended to run for two years and end in January 2023. During this period the firm controversially made a cash donation of £20,000 to Liam Fox.

On 1 June 2022, Fox received the large sum; he then subsequently reported it to the Electoral Commission in late July 2022 and this was then subsequently published in the MPs' register of interest in August 2022.[51][52]

On discovery of the dubious donation to Fox and the previous lobbying by Fox on behalf of SureScreen, Good Law Project collaborated with Phil Kemp at the BBC to reveal to the public what was going on behind closed doors. The news caused quite the stir and was subsequently picked up by most major newspapers.[53]

SureScreen responded to the BBC by claiming that they were not aware "Mr Fox had been in touch with Mr Hancock in 2020"; furthermore they said the £20,000 donation was for "Dr Fox's office – not Dr Fox personally". SureScreen also claimed the donation "was made by one of the directors of the business. This donation was specifically to support a series of events which include education talks from expert guests. The payment is not connected in any way to lobbying." Fox claimed it was a "baseless smear concocted" by Good Law Project.[54]

The following month, in October 2022, a close connection of Fox's was linked to SureScreen. Good Law Project had seen a "series of messages, sent over the course of two years" involving the negotiation of sales for SureScreen products and the involvement of Adam Werrity in that process.[55]

Adam Werritty and Liam Fox are long-term friends; according to reports Werritty was Fox's "best man, a former flatmate and a one-time business partner". In 2011 the pair's close relationship exploded into the news – forcing Fox to resign as defence secretary.[56]

It was reported that Fox and Werritty met on 18 separate overseas trips and a further 22 visits to his MoD office during Fox's tenure as the defence minister ending in 2011, with Werritty organising a meeting between the minister and a defence contractor during one overseas trip – all despite not holding any official role within government or receiving any formal security clearance.

Werritty even went as far as printing and handing out business cards that bear the logo of the Houses of Parliament and carrying the job title of "advisor to the Rt Hon Dr Fox MP".[57]

The political fallout from the Werrity lobbying scandal was huge and ultimately forced Fox to resign from his ministerial position. In his October 2011 resignation letter Fox reflected on his relationship with Werritty, noting: "I mistakenly allowed the distinction between my personal interest and my government activities to become blurred. The consequences of this have become clearer in recent days. I am very sorry for this. I have also repeatedly said that the national interest must always come before personal interest. I now have to hold myself to my own standard. I have therefore decided, with great sadness, to resign from my post as secretary of state for defence – a position which I have been immensely proud and honoured to have held".[58]

When Good Law Project approached SureScreen for comment regarding its relationship with Werritty, the firm's director David Campbell confirmed his company had entered into a contractual relationship with Werritty.

Campbell also confirmed, "During the pandemic, Mr Werrity approached SureScreen via his company to discuss export opportunities. As part of these discussions, he signed our terms and conditions and asked for samples of our tests to be exported for evaluation. Only one of these opportunities, a German company, ever came to fruition and they purchased a small number of tests. The relevant contract was a direct one negotiated between and entered into by SureScreen and the German company only, and not with Mr Werrity".

Following Campbell's comments and shortly before Good Law Project was due to publish its report, a letter marked "Private and Confidential" and "Not for Publication" from SureScreen's lawyers Taylor Wessing landed in the Good Law Project in-tray. SureScreen wanted the story closed down, but Good Law Project pressed ahead. Rightly so. The story was clearly of high public interest.[59]

Thriva

Another company with close ties to the Conservative Party that also benefited from the VIP lane was Thriva Ltd, a private healthcare firm, based at the trendy White Collar Factory in Shoreditch, East London – a modern office skyscraper with its own rooftop running track and commanding views across the city.

Thriva landed two huge government contracts courtesy of the priority route. The first, valued at £61.7 million, was awarded on 10 August 2020 and required Thriva to source components for and subsequently build and deliver testing kits.[60]

A representative from Thriva had held a meeting with health minister and Tory peer Lord Bethell to discuss "Covid-19 testing" in June 2020, three months prior to the first contract award.[61]

The first contract was followed by a second, much larger one the following year, in July 2021, when the DHSC awarded the firm a £124.4 million contract to "provide a comprehensive, end-to-end capillary blood testing service" that would detect the presence of antibodies generated by Covid.[62]

Sandwiched between the two DHSC contracts, Thriva also landed a place, alongside the 49 other suppliers on Public Health England's monstrous £15 billion, two-year-long "diagnostic testing services" framework agreement that would allow public sector bodies to procure testing and laboratory services from the named suppliers – although it's unclear if the firm subsequently landed any contracts from the arrangement.[63]

The contracts were highly profitable for Thriva, whose fortunes turned from a loss in 2020 to recording gross profits of £38.8m by December 2021. Thriva noted in their company accounts filed on Companies House that the "strong performance" was "driven by a mix of growth from Covid-19 related at home testing and non-Covid-19 at home testing". The following year, in December 2022, the firm recorded a further £13.6m in gross profits.[64]

Thriva has strong roots back to a number of senior and influential figures within the Conservative Party.

Firstly, a major shareholder in Thriva is the London-based investment firm Pembroke Venture Capital Trust. Pembroke is chaired by the former Conservative MP for Huntingdon and former justice minister, Jonathan Djanogly.[65]

Djanogly, who first registered his role at Pembroke in 2015, was rewarded well for his work at the investment firm. An investigation I worked on with the David Rose at the *Daily Mail* revealed he was being paid £30,000 per year by the firm for completing approximately 32 hours' work – earning nearly £1,000 per hour.[66]

The founder and current chief executive officer of Pembroke is Andrew Wolfson – his brother Lord Simon Wolfson is a Tory peer and major donor to the Conservative Party as well as a shareholder of Pembroke Venture Capital.[67][68]

Closer to home, Thriva currently has two Conservative peers sitting on its board of directors, both of whom have potentially conflicting links back to the UK government.

Firstly, Tory peer Baroness Blackwood is the current chair of Thriva's advisory board (having been appointed in December 2022). Blackwood served as the MP for Oxford West and Abingdon between 2010 and 2017; she was also a health minister between July 2016 and July 2017. More recently Blackwood has been the chair of Genomics England – a role she has held since May 2020.[69][70]

Secondly, in February 2023, Thriva announced it had appointed Lord James O'Shaughnessy to its advisory board. The Tory peer, like Blackwood, was also a former health minister. During the pandemic O'Shaughnessy worked as an advisor to government health minister Lord Bethell – the role according to O'Shaughnessy involved "providing policy advice to DHSC ministers and officials around testing innovation". The peer's role raised a number of eyebrows when it was first revealed in the press, prompting an investigation by the Public Relations and Communications Association (PRCA) into Portland Communications where O'Shaughnessy previously worked as a consultant.[71][72][73][74]

According to the disclosure provided by the UKHSA in December 2022, Thriva secured its place on the VIP lane by self-referring.[75]

Immensa Health

It wasn't just politically connected Covid testing manufacturers that received the VIP treatment – private sector providers of laboratories also became benefactors of the priority lane.

The government's Test and Trace programme urgently needed lab facilities and their staff to enable the ramping-up of testing capacity. One provider – Immensa Health, owned by Dante Labs – was a big winner of contracts via this route. The British public, however, would have to live with the disastrous consequences of the government's decision to prioritise Immensa's offer.

On 4 September 2020, the DHSC's Test and Trace team entered into a contract with Immensa; the initial contract value was for £119 million and would run until 4 March 2021. In return for the lucrative sum, Immensa was required to conduct PCR testing at its Wolverhampton lab. It was also contracted to conduct PCR testing at an Italian lab run by the firm's parent company, Dante Labs. The contract was awarded without any formal competitive tendering process.[76][77]

It would take a further four months before the first Covid samples were finally sent to Immensa's laboratory in Wolverhampton – and within two weeks of this date, on 31 January 2021, reports of unsafe and negligent working practices began to emerge from the lab.

A damning report in the *Sun on Sunday* newspaper showed undercover footage from inside Immensa's Wolverhampton facility. Workers, wearing the typical long white lab coats, were seen brawling inside and outside the lab, sleeping at their desks, playing football and bragging about drinking Jägermeister while on shift.[78]

The following month, on 24 February 2021, the Welsh government flagged concerns to the DHSC's Test and Trace programme over the quality of results coming from PCR tests analysed at Immensa's laboratory. The Welsh Test, Trace and Protect (TTP) team were concerned about the what they perceived to be an "unusually high positivity rate in results" from tests completed by care home staff in North Wales and processed by Immensa. Public Health Wales (PHW) told the Welsh government: "The above observations raise significant concerns about a range of laboratory processes (including quality control of output) at the Immensa lab, which may be leading to inaccurate results." The concerns were dismissed by DHSC Test and Trace in March 2021, who simply "cut and pasted" the Immensa findings and sent them back to the Welsh government.[79]

Immensa's first contract concluded in March 2021, but according to the UKHSA they were still processing Covid tests up to 12 May 2021.

Despite the serious concerns flagged by the press and the Welsh government regarding Immensa's Wolverhampton lab, the firm landed a second contract in July 2021 to continue PCR testing at the same facility. The deal was valued at an additional £50 million – bringing the total contract value across both deals to £169 million.[80]

Following the second contract award in July 2021, Covid tests started to arrive at Immensa Wolverhampton lab on 2 September 2021. Almost immediately things descended into chaos again, but this time with potentially deadly consequences.

Within six days of testing recommencing at Wolverhampton a strange pattern started to emerge. On 8 September 2021, a resident in Bristol had tested positive for Covid after taking a lateral flow test. However they subsequently tested negative on a PCR test analysed at Immensa lab. An almost identical issue was recorded by a resident in Swindon on 13 September 2021. Soon the floodgates opened and a significant number of people were raising concerns, after being incorrectly told by Immensa their PCR tests were Covid negative when in fact they were positive and carrying the virus.

The scale of Immensa's faulty testing was colossal. Between 2 September 2021 and 12 October 2021 the firm "undertook 417,000 PCR tests" and the UKHSA estimated that circa 43,000 of these tests were incorrectly given as negative results, an estimate it subsequently revised down to 39,000.[81]

The UKHSA eventually suspended operations at Immensa's Wolverhampton lab on 15 October 2021. But this was the equivalent of closing the stable door after the horse had bolted, because the firm's failures had now fed into a spike in Covid cases in the south-west of the country – a catastrophic failure that led to potentially 55,000 additional infections, countless hospital admissions and the avoidable death of up to 23 people, according to the UKHSA.[82]

Exactly how Immensa was able to bag a place on the VIP lane remains unclear. Data handed over to me by the UKHSA following my FOI victory claims the firm simply "self-referred to online portal" and this was their pathway onto the priority route, but this only explains part of the process. For example, who was the official who identified the Immensa offer in the "online portal" and then subsequently fast-tracked them through the VIP lane?

Maybe the UK Covid Inquiry or a future investigation can shine more light onto this case.[83]

Gaps in the data

When the UK government finally disclosed the names of the VIP testing firms and the names of the politicians who referred them in December 2022, it quickly became apparent that the information provided contained a number of gaps, which may have been honest mistakes or potentially could have been deliberate attempts by officials to protect the names of politically linked companies and individuals.

There were examples where UKHSA would state the VIP supplier was identified by a "third party" or a supplier miraculously "self-referred" its bid to an email address that only ministers, MPs and senior officials knew existed.[84]

Additionally the data provided in the December 2022 FOI response only covered 'VIP' suppliers who were awarded contracts after 28 May 2020, despite the priority channels being in existence from March 2020.

I decided to continue digging and soon uncovered a host of new VIP suppliers and further fingerprints of senior Conservative Party figures.

Lord Feldman and Abbott Rapid Diagnostics

Abbott Rapid Diagnostics is a subsidiary of the American multinational healthcare company Abbott Laboratories. It has a long, established history of manufacturing goods in the UK that dates back to 1937, and the firm supplied anaesthetics to the Allied forces during the Second World War.[85]

During the pandemic, Abbott unsurprisingly was able to secure a number of multi-million pound contracts from the government to provide Covid testing kits and laboratory services; however, the relationship got off to an unusual start.

On 25 March 2020 the DHSC awarded a £62.5 million

contract to Abbott to supply "rapid antibody test kits". In an unusual step, the government didn't issue Abbott with a formal contract to execute, it instead signed a "quotation acceptance form" prepared by the supplier. But, before any goods were purchased, the government cancelled the order.[86][87]

Following the failed first contract, Abbott held a meeting with Cabinet minister Lord Agnew on 2 April 2020 to discuss Covid testing. This was followed up by another meeting with health minister Lord Bethell on 7 April 2020 – also in attendance during the meeting was Conservative peer Lord Andrew Feldman.[88][89]

When Shadow Cabinet minister Rachel Hopkins MP asked health minister Edward Argar for details of the meeting between Abbott, Lord Bethell and Lord Feldman, she was told controversially that the DHSC didn't take any minutes of the meeting.

Argar told the Labour MP: "The Department does not hold a formal minute of the meeting. Lord Bethell attended the meeting with a Private Secretary, officials from the Department and the Medicines and Healthcare products Regulatory Authority, Lord Feldman of Elstree and representatives from Abbott. Special advisors did not attend the meeting. Lord Feldman of Elstree attended in an advisory capacity."[90]

Following the meeting with ministers, Abbott developed and offered another Covid test to the UK government – the Panbio Covid-19 Antigen Rapid Test Device – and on 11 September 2020, health officials placed a £44 million contract with Abbott to begin supplying the new test in bulk.[91]

A month later, on 7 October 220, the DHSC increased its order with Abbott and purchased further Covid tests from the firm valued at an additional £120 million. From there on Abbott steadily picked up further contracts from the UK government and by September 2021 had been paid £305 million by the government to provide medical goods.[92]

Abbott was a beneficiary of the VIP lane. It secured its place after a "third party" contacted Lord Bethell.[93]

I wanted to know who this mysterious third party was, so in early December 2023, I asked the UKHSA via a FOI request to provide that person's name. Four months of stonewalling later, the government body finally responded: "I can confirm that the third party referred to in your request is Andrew Feldman".

It was now clear that Lord Feldman had not only referred PPE suppliers on to the VIP lane (see Chapter 1), but that he was also identifying potential VIPs for the Test and Trace programme.

I discussed earlier in this chapter how Dominic Cummings claimed Rishi Sunak's team worked with him to "secretly buy hundreds of millions of fast tests" and overcome Whitehall bureaucracy. According to health officials, Abbott, alongside Innova Medical, was a supplier of the tests Cummings was referring to.

An FOI response from the UKHSA confirmed it was Abbott's 11 September 2020 contract to supply £44 million worth of Covid tests that picked up the attention of Cummings. A review of the government spending data during this period revealed the DHSC paid Abbott £11.3 million over a four-day period between 10 and 14 September 2020. The payments were broken down into 192 separate transactions and labelled with the description "Testing kits".

Interestingly, I would later discover the government deliberately edited out Lord Feldman's name from the disclosure published on the VIP lane. An email I obtained via FOI request and sent between civil servants on 19 December 2020, just two days before they published the VIP list, reads: "I've removed the identity of the third party for Abbott so we are consistent in our references (Good Law Project can FOI us if needed…)"

The missing VIPs

The disclosure of 50 VIP firms by the UKHSA in December 2022 only covered referrals post 28 May 2020. However, the fast-track lane was in operation from 15 March 2020, possibly earlier.

A day after the UKHSA responded with the VIP names, I asked them to confirm how many other companies were referred onto the high-priority route from mid-March 2020 up to the end of May 2020.

In January 2023, health officials responded to my request and confirmed the names of two additional suppliers who met the 'priority' criteria. In its response UKHSA judged the suppliers on the following metric:

"Suppliers were investigated further as their correspondence referred to one of the following criteria, and then went on to be awarded a contract by DHSC:

1. "VIP" "FASTTRACK" "High Priority" and "Referral" mentioned in correspondence

2. Suppliers involved in email correspondence with a "VIP" individual ("ps-", "@parliament" or "No10" email addresses)

3. Involved in correspondence via the "priority contacts" mailbox."

The two new names were Nationwide Pathology Ltd, which was awarded a contract to conduct PCR testing following a referral from its local Tory MP Alberto Costa, who subsequently contacted secretary of state Matt Hancock on the firm's behalf on 26 March 2020. The second supplier was Perkinelmer Las (UK) Ltd, which won VIP contracts to supply PCR testing services and laboratory equipment.

The pandemic years proved to be incredibly fruitful for Nationwide and its directors. The firm's turnover increased dramatically between 2020 and 2022 due to the "company's significant involvement in the UK's international arrivals scheme". Furthermore Nationwide claimed it had become "one of the largest suppliers of Covid testing to UKHSA throughout the pandemic".[94]

Nationwide's annual accounts filed with Companies House certainly supported this claim. Over a two-year period that ended 31 March 2022 the firm had recorded a turnover of £86 million and a healthy gross profit of £46 million.

Nationwide's business model was heavily reliant on the Covid testing; this was demonstrated when the VIP firm published its accounts covering the first year after the pandemic. Turnover dropped from £58 million down to £5 million. The significant drop in business led to the directors laying off staff and mothballing its "mass testing equipment".

Nationwide Pathology is controlled by the Dunn family, who are also the firm's directors. During the company's bumper two years in the midst of the pandemic, they rewarded themselves with dividend payouts of £13 million.

In 2022 and 2023, Jamie and Sheryl Dunn started to spend their vast sums of wealth generated during the pandemic. Documents obtained from the HM Land Registry confirm the pair spent £8 million in February 2022 purchasing a huge piece of land from the Thorpe Lubenham Hall estate in North-amptonshire. The pair were also granted planning permission to build a new four-bed home as well as a huge new laboratory on land formerly owned by the estate.[95][96]

Randox Laboratories Ltd and Owen Paterson

If you scroll down the list of 50 VIPs declared by the UKHSA, you will notice one obvious candidate for the high-priority route appears to be missing – Randox Laboratories Ltd.[97]

The government's pandemic contracts with Randox proved to be highly controversial and politically sensitive – the huge public outcry once details of the contracts finally started to emerge was of a scale second only to Baroness Mone and the PPE Medpro deals (discussed in Chapter 1).

According to the NAO, which conducted an investigation into the Randox contracts in March 2022, health officials told them Randox were not identified as high-priority suppliers.

The NAO said: "Officials told us they do not consider that Randox came through the test and trace procurement high-priority entry routes created early in the pandemic to deal with supplier referrals from 'high-ranked individuals' such as ministers, MPs and the Prime Minister's Office. The analysis that UKHSA conducted retrospectively in January 2022 to identify high-priority suppliers focused on activity from May 2020 to March 2021, two months after the award of Randox's first testing contract".[98]

The retrospective analysis referred to by the NAO was problematic; as I discussed earlier in the chapter, it failed to capture contracts placed prior to May 2020. Randox was awarded its first deal on 30 March 2020.[99]

However, one name that does appear on the VIP list is Qnostics Ltd. According to the Glasgow-based firm's website, it is a "leading provider of Quality Control Solutions for molecular infectious disease testing". Qnostics is ultimately controlled by Dr Peter FitzGerald.[100]

Dr Peter FitzGerald is also the ultimate controlling party for another company – Randox.[101]

In fact, the ties between Randox and Qnostics are incredibly close, almost indistinguishable. Not only do they share the same owner, but they also previously shared the same director – chartered accountant Richard Kelly. Furthermore, Qnostics' website consists of a page on the Randox.com website and, most revealing, the two companies were considered to be "strategic partners" by government officials, who subsequently awarded 22 contracts valued at £776.9 million.[102][103]

So how did this partnership led by Randox manage to secure so many Covid contracts? The answer involves a "consultant" who was also a serving Conservative Party MP at the time, a handful of government ministers and a huge lobbying scandal that ultimately forced the release of key correspondence covering the months before and after the contracts were awarded.

On the 26 January 2020, the Conservative MP for North Shropshire, Owen Paterson, reached out to the secretary of state Matt Hancock. Paterson contacted Hancock at his personal email address. Within four minutes of receiving the email Hancock replied to Paterson and within ten minutes Hancock subsequently contacted the Randox director, Peter FitzGerald, as per Paterson's request.[104]

The initial emails between Paterson and Hancock were short but direct:

Owen Paterson, 26/01/2020, 21:23: "Thanks call Peter FitzGerald's email: [Redacted]@randox.com if you can get ten positive sputum samples, they will take 2-3 weeks to develop a diagnostic test giving results for coronavirus within 23 hours based on raw sputum samples."

Matt Hancock, 26/01/2020, 21:27: "Thanks Owen. I will look into it."

Owen Paterson, 26/01/2020, 21:29: "Thanks. Have told him to expect an email from you. Ring anytime if you want to discuss."

Matt Hancock's email to Peter FitzGerald read: "Hi Peter, Thanks for getting in touch. I understand that if you can get positive sputum samples, you will be able to develop a diagnostic test within a number of weeks giving results for coronavirus within 2/3 hours based on raw sputum samples. I would be grateful for more detail so we can look into it. Matt."

Paterson's lobbying on behalf of Randox was already under the spotlight at this point, after it was revealed in 2019 that the Tory MP had held several meetings with officials and a minister on behalf of two firms – Lynn County Foods and Randox. Paterson had declared in the register of members' financial interests that he was being paid £8,333 a month by Randox for 16 hours' work each month; however, prior to taking up the role Paterson informed officials his work wouldn't involve lobbying the government on behalf of the firm.[105][106]

The NAO noted in its investigation that Paterson "sought advice on taking up his Randox role from the Advisory Committee on Business Appointments (the Committee), given the former ministerial positions he held from 2010 to 2014" and the committee subsequently confirmed: "Although Randox will have engagement with government in pursuit of its business, you have informed us that it will not be part of your role with the company to be involved in such engagement". Paterson's lobbying of ministers and "egregious" breach of the rule would later be responsible for ending his parliamentary career.[107][108]

By January 2020, Randox had also handed £160,000 in cash

donations to the Conservative Party, over an eight-year period starting in 2010.[109]

On 27 January 2020, the day following Paterson's initial lobbying of Matt Hancock, the owner of Randox Peter FitzGerald got in touch with Hancock. He was keen to progress the development of the Randox Covid test and needed ten positive samples from the government to aid with the development of the device. Later the same day Hancock forwarded the request from FitzGerald on to the chief medical officer's office.

Throughout February Paterson continued to pepper Matt Hancock via WhatsApp messages, chasing up progress on behalf of Randox. One such message sent on 25 February 2020 read: "It is now 19 days since PHE last contacted Randox at your request. Since then EVAg have provided a positive sample and the Randox test worked perfectly. Test kits are now being shipped to China, Mexico, Ukraine, Oman, Tunisia and Guatemala. PHE's attitude looks incomprehensible given current developments and time pressures. Are you voting today? Can we discuss briefly? Great announcement on pharmacies by the way! Best wishes. Owen". Hancock promptly forwarded the message on to officials, urging PHE to "get on this".

By March 2020, the Randox and UK government relationship was growing stronger and an email from civil servants to Matt Hancock on 1 March 2020 confirmed that the Randox offering had been "prioritised".[110]

On 17 March 2020 Randox attended a round-table meeting to discuss Covid-19 mass testing headed up by Prime Minister Boris Johnson and with Matt Hancock and a group of other suppliers in attendance. The following day, 18 March 2020, Randox attended another meeting, this time organised by health minister Lord Bethell. Bethell would later be criticised for failing to declare Randox's attendance at the meeting – a key transparency rule that the minister failed to comply with on four separate occasions during his dealings with Randox and Paterson.

According to officials speaking to the NAO, the 18 March 2020 meeting with Bethell was crucial for Randox and led to "to contractual negotiations with the company to establish the number of tests that Randox could deliver per day, the cost per test and any support that it might need to fulfil its contractual commitments". Although when the NAO asked the DHSC to provide further details of the negotiations it was unable to provide any supporting information.[111]

Just six days later, on 24 March 2020, Bethell approved the first deal with Randox and the contract was formally issued on 30 March 2020. The government committed itself to purchasing 2.7 million tests from Randox at an eye-watering cost of £49.26 each. The initial contract value was agreed at £133 million and included an upfront payment of £50 million as "security for their commitment". The contract was also awarded without any formal competitive tendering process.[112]

The first contact between Randox and the UK government got off to a rocky start, and Randox struggled to obtain enough specialist laboratory equipment required to ramp up testing capacity, partly due to factors outside its control, and throughout the April to September 2020 period it was consistently completing lower numbers of tests than had been set out in the contract.

On 15 July 2020, the contract came under further scrutiny, as it emerged the Medicines and Healthcare products Regulatory Agency (MHRA) had issued a major recall of the Randox home testing kit after the swabs included with the device failed to "required safety standards for coronavirus testing" – up to

750,000 unused tests were recalled from members of the public and care homes.[113][114]

Two and half months after the mass recall of tests, on 2 October 2020, Randox was directly awarded with a further contract from the UK government to continue Covid testing until the end of March 2021. The value of the award was huge – £328.3 million.[115][116]

In the build-up to the October contract award, concerns were raised by Cabinet Office minister Lord Agnew, who said on 25 September 2020: "I'm very worried about pricing. Given the huge volumes we are paying dramatically over the odds".

The same day, further concerns were also echoed by the Cabinet Office permanent secretary, Alex Chisholm, who said: "I am disappointed that despite entering into the original contract on 30 March DHSC have not moved to organise and conclude a competitive contract process and are now in a position where extension by direct award is the only viable option. Can we please insist on a written commitment from DHSC to initiate a competitive process in time for new contracts to be let from March 2021. At least the price has been negotiated down and is now comparable to benchmarks, and quality has been good."[117]

The concerns flagged by Agnew and Chisolm did lead to additional measures being included in the contract, but nonetheless it didn't stop the award to Randox, which a month later was again cast into the spotlight for all the wrong reasons.

In November 2020, Channel 4's *Dispatches* aired its new documentary titled 'Lockdown Chaos: How the Government Lost Control'. The documentary makers broadcasted undercover footage from inside Randox's testing facility in Northern Ireland. According to Channel 4 the film provided evidence of "Covid tests being accidentally discarded, tests leaking out of vials, and the potential of cross-contamination of tests that could potentially lead to individuals getting the wrong test results."[118]

In response to the documentary, Randox initially disputed the findings, claiming they were "underhand, deceptive, dishonest and defamatory". However, the Health and Safety Executive Northern Ireland (HSENI) saw enough evidence to warrant a site visit to the Randox lab and immediately directed the firm to "take immediate action to address significant safety concerns, both Covid-19-related and general, observed at the site", according to the NAO findings.[119]

Throughout the course of the pandemic the UK government awarded 22 contracts and contract variations to Randox and its strategic partner Qnostics. The awards had a combined value of 776.9 million, of which Randox had been paid £403 million by October 2021. This created huge profits for the firm.

In the 18 months up to June 2020 Randox reported a loss of £12 million, but following the contract award the company's fortunes changed dramatically and by June 2021, Randox Holdings Ltd recorded profits before tax of £275 million – record profits for the firm.[120][121]

The following year, covering the period up to June 2022, the firm reported additional profits of £190 million. In two years Randox had generated £465 million in profit.[122]

The fallout from the government's dealing with Randox and Owen Paterson was huge. Boris Johnson was forced into spending weeks defending claims of sleaze and corruption at the heart of his administration.

When Boris Johnson failed to get to grips with the unravelling scandal or apologise for the governments conduct, the then leader of the opposition Sir Keir Starmer accused the PM of being a "coward" and further claimed he was giving "the green light for corruption".[123]

When it was discovered that ministers had not kept any meeting minutes of discussions with Randox and Paterson, the shadow deputy leader Angela Rayner took to social media to call out the perceived "corruption". She wrote: "A government minister just confirmed in Parliament that there are no minutes to the meeting(s) that took place between Lord Bethell, Owen Paterson and Randox as part of Randox being awarded £600 million of contracts without any kind of tender or any process. This is corruption.

"By admitting that no minutes exist for the Randox lobbying meetings, the government has admitted that the government is routinely breaking the Ministerial Code. When a minister meets an organisation or company an official must be present to keep a record of that meeting."[124]

On 26 October 2021, the parliamentary commissioner for standards published their findings following an inquiry into Owen Paterson's lobbying activity. It determined that "Mr Paterson's actions, in particular those relating to paid advocacy, constitute a serious breach of the rules".

Furthermore, the committee found "Mr Paterson's actions were an egregious case of paid advocacy, that he repeatedly used his privileged position to benefit two companies for whom he was a paid consultant, and that this has brought the House into disrepute."

The committee noted that they hadn't previously encountered a case of paid lobbying which had seen so many breaches of the rules, which spanned from 2016 to 2020.

Paterson breached the MPs' code of conduct, paragraph 11 (which prohibits paid advocacy), on multiple occasions relating to his role with Randox. Furthermore Paterson breached paragraph 15 of the MPs' code of conduct when he facilitated 25 business meetings with his clients from his parliamentary office. A week after the report was published, Paterson resigned as a member of Parliament.[125]

In July 2022, the House of Commons Committee of Public Accounts published its findings following an investigation into the government's contracts with Randox. It concluded the DHSC's record-keeping was "woefully inadequate" and that it had failed to meet basic transparency requirements relating to ministerial meetings with Randox. Furthermore and despite clear concerns with Randox's political connection the department failed to deal with the potential "conflict of interest".

The committee was also scathing over the award of the contracts, which it believed "did not receive adequate scrutiny from senior officials and the role of ministers in signing it was unclear". It was also extremely critical over the failure by officials to hold Randox to account for its performance in the initial contract and the decision to award the firm with another £328m contract without competition. Randox's record-breaking profits also came under the glare of the committee, which suggested the government should "strengthen its commercial guidance on ensuring profits are not excessive".[126]

In October 2022, following a four-year pause, Randox resumed handing cash donations to the Conservative Party. Firstly with a £8,800 donation in 2022, followed by two £6,300 donations in 2023, increasing the total amount handed to the Tories to £182,200.[127]

When the dust finally settled on the government's flagship Covid programme, the taxpayer was left to foot a £29.5 billion bill for the highly inefficient Test and Trace programme, which enriched many politically connected companies with huge paydays but ultimately failed to achieve its main objective of avoiding further national lockdowns and breaking the chain of transmission.[128]

Tanner Pharma – tracking down the new VIPs

Nearly five years after the first case of Covid-19 in the UK, still the public did not have the complete picture regarding the true scale of the Test and Trace VIP lane. In December 2024, after another lengthy transparency battle with the UK Health Security Agency, I was able to reveal the names of another two VIP suppliers – whose names remain missing from the data published by the health department.

Those new VIP suppliers were Source Bioscience UK limited and Tanner Pharma UK Limited. The latter immediately jumped out of the screen at me and grabbed my attention. I had previously reported on this company and its owner, the American banker Raymond Fairbanks Bourne – often referred to as Banks Bourne.

In October 2023, more than a year prior to UKHSA coming clean over Tanner's VIP status, I had reported that Mr Bourne had paid himself handsomely following the success of Tanner's government contracts. In total Mr Banks paid himself £149 million in dividends via the Tanner Pharma UK business – the firm's Covid contracts during this period accounted for the majority of its turnover and profit.

I noted Banks Bourne, the sole director and owner of Tanner Pharma UK, had for the second year running paid himself a staggering £76m in dividends; this followed a £73m payment the previous year.

In total Mr Bourne has received over £149m in dividend payments since the firm secured multiple and highly lucrative Covid testing contracts from the Department of Health and Social Care in 2020 and 2021.

According to data compiled by Tussell, Tanner Pharma UK was awarded nine contracts from the UK government to provide lateral flow devices valued at up to £1.45 billion, resulting in £180m gross profits for the firm to date.

Tanner Pharma UK's turnover is almost entirely reliant on the UK government. Approximately 97% of the company's turnover was generated from its Covid deals in the UK, according to records published on Companies House.

In the US, Bourne and Tanner Pharma UK's eye-watering contracts with the UK government are at the centre of an ongoing multimillion-dollar lawsuit.

According to reports, "A lawsuit filed in the Charlotte federal courts accuses the former Wachovia investment banker, his pharmaceutical-supply companies, and a top associate of improperly withholding hundreds of millions of dollars in profits that were owed to a business partner".

Furthermore, a report published by Good Law Project revealed Tanner Pharma was one of six companies that provided unusable Covid tests to the Department of Health and Social Care during the pandemic. In total the six firms provided £246 million in unusable goods. Tanner Pharma UK claims it is not aware of any kits being rejected by authorities in the UK.

Tanner Pharma UK was not the only Covid testing firm to make huge profits from contracts secured under the government's controversial Test and Trace programme.

A spokesperson for Tanner Pharma UK said:

"Tanner Pharma UK Limited earned contracts from the DHSC to provide lateral flow Covid-19 tests for use in the United Kingdom. These tests were selected because, when evaluated at Porton Down, they were determined to have both very high specificity and very high sensitivity against viral loads associated with infectiousness. We are proud to have successfully delivered over 480 million reliable, accurate testing kits as part of the emergency response to the pandemic.

"At all times, Tanner Pharma UK Limited acted within its contractual rights, and generously compensated FS Medical Supplies. Their claims in the lawsuit in the US are without merit, and some claims have already been dismissed by the Court. We remain confident in our case."

Ironically, the latest accounts published by Tanner in December 2024 have shown turnover at Tanner Pharma UK has declined by 96% since the UK government stopped procuring Covid tests from them and operating profit plummeted from £67m in 2022 to a loss of £9 million in 2023.[129]

We now know that the £1.4 billion worth of Covid testing contracts awarded to Tanner, which led to the £149 million in dividend rewards being paid to Banks Bourne, were facilitated by the company's inclusion in the VIP lane – something to this day the government has not directly declared to the British public.[130]

Chapter 3

The peers

During the pandemic the Conservative-led government frequently recruited personnel for high-profile and highly critical roles from a small pool of candidates – the pool was the House of Lords and the candidates were often Conservative Party peers.

Not only did the government close ranks for Tory-linked firms who they subsequently enabled via the VIP lane, bestowing those companies with unimaginable wealth (as seen in Chapters 1 and 2), they also ensured Conservative Party politicians were drafted in to lead the flagship programmes responsible for handing out those lucrative contracts.

Baroness Dido Harding was hired by Prime Minister Boris Johnson to run the NHS Test and Trace programme. Lord James Bethell was promoted to health minister by Matt Hancock in March 2020. Bethell had previously led Matt Hancock's failed leadership campaign in 2019 and had also donated £5,000 to Hancock and a further £5,000 into the Tory coffers during the same period.[1]

Conservative peers Lord Andrew Feldman and Lord James

O'Shaughnessy were also appointed as key advisors to health ministers during the first wave of the pandemic in spring 2020 – despite Feldman's potential conflicts of interests (again see Chapters 1 and 2).

Boris Johnson was also responsible for appointing another Tory peer into an influential role. In April 2020, Lord Paul Deighton was appointed the government's new PPE Tzar – a role that saw him oversee the procurement of PPE, including contracts that operated via the VIP lane.

Lord Deighton – PPE Tzar

On 17 April 2020, Boris Johnson's chief of staff, Edward Lister – now Lord Udny-Lister – spoke with Lord Deighton. The same evening he shared the news via a WhatsApp message to No. 10 colleagues: "Spoke to Paul Deighton tonight and gave him my less than kind take on PPE. I know him of old he will be good at this". Two days later Deighton was appointed by the PM to lead the PPE programme.[2]

Deighton is a former investment banker at Goldman Sachs. Between 2013 and 2015 he served as the commercial secretary to the Treasury, under David Cameron's premiership having previously been the chief executive of the London Organising Committee of the Olympic and Paralympic Games (LOCOG), the organisers responsible for the planning of the London 2012 Olympic and Paralympic games.[3]

Deighton was appointed to lead the PPE procurement drive despite a number of obvious conflicts of interest. In December 2020, following an investigation by the *New York Times*, a large spotlight was shone on Deighton's conflicting financial interests.

The New York Times discovered Deighton remained "involved in business and has financial or personal connections to at least seven companies that were awarded lucrative government contracts totalling nearly $300 million".[4]

Honeywell Safety Products, a subsidiary of Honeywell International, a company Deighton held shares in during the pandemic, was awarded a £57.9 million PPE contract to supply face masks – a deal awarded without any formal competitive tendering process.[5]

In March 2025, a document published by the Covid Inquiry revealed that Lord Deighton held a meeting with "senior" representatives from Honeywell to discuss the firm's face mask deal on 27 April 2020. Just ten days later Honeywell secured its bumper PPE contract to supply the same masks.

Lord Deighton confirmed in his witness statement issued to the Covid Inquiry that "on 27 April 2020, I held a senior meeting with Honeywell to discuss the high-level plans which were then passed to procurement teams for review".

The statement also confirms that Deighton was involved in correspondence regarding the "price comparison" of the masks being offered by Honeywell. The Conservative Peer did discuss his investment in Honeywell with senior civil servants, but it was concluded "there would be no conflict, given the relatively small contracts would not move the share price of such a large company".

Deighton also denied any involvement in approving the contract to Honeywell.

On 4 May 2020, Deighton's register of interest held by the House of Lords was updated and a new shareholding in AstraZeneca was revealed. Just a week previously, on 27 April 2020, the British pharmaceutical company was awarded a £152 million contract by the DHSC to provide Covid testing services.[6]

AstraZeneca was also contracted by the UK government to develop and supply the Covid vaccination and by October

2021 40 million doses had been provided by the firm. Deighton only relinquished his shareholdings in the company on 30 June 2023.[7][8]

During his time as PPE Tzar, Deighton also held shares in the consulting firm Accenture and banking firm UBS – both secured Covid-related contracts from the UK government.

Lord Deighton is also chairman and a major shareholder of a secretive intelligence firm called Hakluyt & Company Ltd.

Hakluyt was founded by a former MI6 officer and boasts the former head of GCHQ, Iain Lobban, as an advisor – along with former bosses of multinationals such as HSBC, Rolls-Royce and Unilever.[9]

The company was accused of spying on environmental campaign groups in 2001 to collect information for oil companies including Shell and BP. Its list of clients is kept secret. The company saw revenue grow to a record £67.2 million in June 2020 and by June 2023 turnover had increased again to £113 million – generating gross profits of £97 million.[10]

I discovered Deighton's "spy" firm met with a UK minister in November 2020 to discuss PPE supply.

In a report published for Open Democracy, we revealed the minister for investment, Lord Grimstone, met with Hakluyt & Company Ltd on 19 November 2020. No minutes were taken of the meeting between Grimstone and the firm, which is known as a "retirement home for ex-MI6 officers".

The Department for International Trade has refused to confirm which Hakluyt representatives attended. But internal documents obtained via FOI request show that a government operation called Project DEFEND was discussed at the meeting.

Project DEFEND was established in the early months of the pandemic – reportedly in a bid to reduce the UK's reliance on China for medical equipment, PPE and other essential supplies.[11]

Deighton appointed and surrounded himself with a temporary team of advisors, which included "senior executives from the private sector", to help with the PPE procurement efforts. But when I asked to see a copy of the names of the executives the Department of Health refused my requests made under the FOI Act to reveal their identities. Four years on, those names still remain a secret.

Lord Deighton was also embroiled in the VIP lane saga again in December 2021. When I forced the government to publish the details of the high-priority lane contracts, Deighton's name was on the list. The Conservative party peer's office was named as both the "source" and "actual referrer" of the China-based Wuhan Xiaoyaoyao Pharmaceuticals.[12]

Wuhan Xiaoyaoyao was awarded a £67.3 million contract on 5 June 2020; the deal involved the firm providing 200 million type IIR face masks, manufactured by Chinese manufacturer Puliyan (Nanjing) Medical Technology Company Limited. It's unclear how many of the 200 million masks were delivered under the contract; however, data published by the DHSC confirms a single payment of £61.3 million was paid to Wuhan Xiaoyaoyao in August 2020.

Intrigued by Lord Deighton being named as the "source" of this firm's route onto the VIP lane, and suspicious that an intermediary or broker may have been involved in lobbying the peer, I submitted another FOI request asking for email correspondence between Deighton and Wuhan Xiaoyaoyao.

I quickly encountered my first problem – I didn't know what email address Deighton was using. The Tory Lord had previously been revealed to have used his private email address during the pandemic for government business and when I initially approached the DHSC for a copy of his emails, they promptly replied and said the department does "not hold the information requested".[13]

Eventually government officials confirmed Deighton's email address was "owned" by the Department for Business, Energy and Industrial Strategy (BEIS) and I swiftly presented them with a fresh FOI request.

In January 2024, BEIS replied to my request and provided an email dated 10 May 2020. The email was from an individual called Mehreen Malik to Lord Deighton with the subject header "Sequoia Capital China and Xiaoyaoyao Relationship Statement". Malik was forwarding on a statement from Sequoia Capital revealing they held a 14.64% stake in the parent company of Wuhan Xiaoyaoyao – a firm that Sequoia valued at "beyond 1 billion USD".

Malik informed Deighton that officials "can contact Sequoia anytime for help on the due diligence if needs be". Less than a month after the email was sent, Wuhan Xiaoyaoyao was awarded its £61.3million contract – a deal that was awarded without any formal competitive tendering process.[14]

Sequoia Capital China is a subsidiary of US-based venture capital firm Sequoia Capital, founded in 1973. In October 2022, Lord Deighton's corporate "spy" firm Hakluyt appointed Sequoia's global chief policy officer, Don Viera, to its board of directors. Lord Deighton was pleased with the appointment, noting, "His perspective on key policy issues, and judgement on matters of governance, will be of great value as we continue to support Hakluyt's success and growth."[15][16]

Deighton also found himself caught up in the 'Pandora Papers' scandal in October 2021, when it emerged he had not declared to officials direct shareholdings he held secretly offshore alongside his wife, Alison. The couple held investments in a number of companies but shielded the transactions from public view via a British Virgin Islands-based venture fund managed by a company called Dawn Capital.[17]

Deighton was far from the only lord to hold questionable investments. During the pandemic prominent Conservative peers frequently became linked to companies earning a fortune out of the pandemic – take for example the former health minister Lord Markham.

Lord Markham and Cignpost Diagnostics

In September 2022, the DHSC appointed Lord Markham CBE as its new parliamentary undersecretary of state. The Tory peer's ministerial portfolio included taking on responsibility for the department's data and technology programmes, procurement issues and among other things cost recovery and fraud prevention.

Prior to this appointment, Nicholas Markham held a number of non-executive board member roles within government. To facilitate his promotion to health minister, Markham was made a life peer by Prime Minister Liz Truss during her turbulent seven-week premiership, taking on the title Baron Markham of East Horsley in the county of Surrey.[18][19]

Markham's appointment to the DHSC came with one glaringly obvious and significant conflict of interest – the Tory peer held a large stake in a government-approved Covid testing company.

Cignpost Diagnostics Limited, a company registered in Farnborough in Hampshire, was incorporated by Markham alongside three other shareholders on 9 June 2020. The firm offered laboratory testing services and established a prominent position providing rapid Covid testing results to travellers flying in and out of Heathrow, Gatwick and Edinburgh Airport – charging £119 per test.[20][21]

The private Covid testing market became very lucrative for Markham and Cignpost and the firm notched up turnover in excess of £44 million and gross profits of £29 million in its first year of trading.[22]

Away from public gaze, Cignpost was busy lobbying politicians and officials. The firm attended two round table meetings hosted by health minister Lord Bethell on 29 April 2021 and 20 August 2021 – the purpose of the meetings was to discuss the "private provider testing market" and "laboratory testing provision for international arrivals" into UK airports – a subject matter that was crucial to Cignpost's continued fortunes.[23][24]

Throughout 2021, Cignpost made proficient use of all-party parliamentary groups (APPGs) inside Westminster to push its Covid testing services.

APPGs are informal, cross-party groups within the UK Parliament that bring together MPs and members of the House of Lords to focus on specific topics or issues. These groups are not official parliamentary committees but function as platforms for parliamentarians to engage with stakeholders, experts and the public on a wide range of policy areas. However, these poorly regulated groups have a dark side.

Critics argue that some APPGs lack transparency in their operations, including funding sources and decision-making processes, potentially raising concerns about undue influence which could create a situation where certain APPGs may be dominated by vested interests, leading to the prioritisation of specific agendas.

Labour MP Chris Bryant, the former chair of the Commons Select Committee on Standards provides a succinct and balanced view regarding both sides of the APPG argument. He points out "all-Party Parliamentary Groups (APPG) may be informal but they provide a great service in the UK's democracy. In good hands, they can foster better relations with other countries or they can keep a weather eye on an authoritarian regime. They can bring into sharp focus a policy issue that might otherwise have been forgotten".

However, on the flip side Bryant highlights the worrying increase in the number of APPGs over recent years, stating "some industries are especially well resourced, with every part of the supply chain and every trade body getting its own group. Some countries have more than one group. We now have more APPGs than we do MPs. It feels as if every MP wants their own APPG and every lobbying company sees an APPG as an ideal way of making a quick buck out of a trade or industry body. 'Look,' the lobbying firms say, 'if you really want to get widgets on the agenda politically, we can get you access to MPs, peers and ministers – but the more financial support you give the APPG (through us, of course) the more effective the group will be.' Hence the rise in the number of APPGs that are serviced by lobbying, PR or communications companies."[25]

Cignpost certainly made keen use of one APPG in particular – the All-Party Parliamentary Group for Business in a Pandemic (Covid) World. The group's purpose was to create a forum where the private sector and politicians could meet and discuss how the "business community" can "continue functioning during a pandemic". Between 21 July 2020 and 20 July 2022, Cignpost funded the APPG's secretariat, donating up to £52,500 to cover its costs.

Cignpost's CEO Steve Whatley was appointed the APPG's "co-chair of the steering committee" and also helped to set up the parliamentary group. Representatives from Cignpost attended and gave presentations to MPs and peers at four out of the first five meetings held by the parliamentary group between September 2020 and January 2021. Markham gave a presentation to politicians at one such event on 26 January 2021.[26][27][28]

Cignpost also donated a further £7,501 to a second parliamentary group – the 'Business Resilience' APPG. The firm's cash covered the admin costs for the group between September 2022 and September 2023.[29]

Cignpost's lobbying efforts didn't end with APPGs. It hired corporate lobbyists Hume Brophy Communications Ltd to lobby government officials on its behalf – a role they fulfilled consistently from July 2021 through to at least October 2022. The director of public affairs at Hume Brophy is Mark MacGregor, the former chief executive officer of the Conservative Party and deputy director of the right-wing think tank the Policy Exchange.[30][31]

Three months after Markham's elevation to the House of Lords, questions started to be raised about the health minister's perceived conflict of interests. Speaking to the *Guardian* newspaper Angela Rayner, Labour deputy leader, said: "Conservative cronies have been rewarded with peerages and plum ministerial jobs while maintaining lucrative interests. There is a rotten stench about the revolving door the Tories have left wide open. Labour will clean up politics by restoring standards in public life with an independent ethics and integrity commission."

The Liberal Democrats piled in too. Sal Brinton, the party's health spokesperson for the House of Lords, said: "These interests are not just inappropriate, but downright unethical. The rules say that ministers should remove any conflicts of interest to prevent any influence on their judgment and maintain the public's trust. Our minister should be held to the highest standards, but these are slipping with each new appointment. Lord Markham should dispose of these interests and Rishi Sunak must immediately appoint a new ethics adviser."[32]

On 25 January 2023, 48 hours after the *Guardian* article was published, Lord Markham tried to tackle the criticisms from across the house head on. He boldly claimed, "I thank the noble Lord. Given the recent press, I want to start by setting out the position of Cignpost, the private sector Covid testing company in which, as many noble Lords will be aware, I own a stake. To be clear, Cignpost did not bid for any government PPE contracts and has only private sector clients. None the less, upon taking up the role as an unpaid Minister of Health, I resigned my directorships, made an undertaking to sell my stake, and in conjunction with the Permanent Secretary, ensured that I was not engaged in any areas where there could be perceived to be a conflict – I just wanted to make that clear".[33]

Markham's plans to divest from Cignpost seemed like the appropriate and principled next step to take, considering the obvious conflict his dual roles represent. However, a year had passed since his pledge, and the Conservative peer had failed to sell his stake; instead he continued to have an interest as the company raked in millions of pounds in profits.

An investigation I conducted with Nick Sommerlad at the *Mirror* discovered that as of January 2024 and one year after Markham told Parliament he would be divesting from the Covid testing firm, he still owned between 25% and 50% of Cignpost Investments Ltd, the parent company of Cignpost Diagnostics. Our investigation discovered Cignpost had filed accounts "showing that revenue soared by 467% to £278 million in 2022, thanks to booming business helping firms comply with Covid rules". Cignpost also held £52 million cash in the bank and its shareholder funds leaped by 150% from the previous year. Cignpost had also pivoted its business to offer mobile health screening, "including heart health assessments and skin screening" – further adding to Markham's conflict of interest.

The DHSC failed to provide an explanation into Markham's lack of action to divest from Cignpost.[34]

At the time of writing in summer 2025, Markham still receives renumeration from Cignpost according to his register of financial interest published by the House of Lords.

Lord Ashcroft and the Covid Vaccine roll-out

The healthcare company ultimately controlled by leading Tory donor and former party chairman Lord Ashcroft received a £350 million contract as part of the government's Covid-19 vaccination rollout, I discovered while freelancing for Peter Geoghegan at Open Democracy.[35]

On 18 December 2020, the DHSC awarded the lucrative contract to Medacs Healthcare plc. Around the same time period the outsourcing company, which specialises in providing staff to the NHS, social care services and private healthcare providers, had been advertising for staff to work on the huge vaccination project.[36]

Medacs is a subsidiary of Impellam Group, a FTSE-listed firm whose largest shareholder is Michael Ashcroft, the Belize-based Conservative peer who has donated millions to the party, including more than £450,000 since the start of 2020. [37]

Ashcroft was non-executive chairman of Impellam and the largest shareholder in the publicly listed company, according to documents filed at Companies House covering the period.

Impellam describes itself as a "leading global talent

acquisition and managed workforce solutions provider". In the two annual reports covering the periods up to January 2021 and December 2021 the firm recorded combined gross profits of £495 million. Its healthcare division, Medacs Healthcare plc recorded profits of £43 million during the same period.[38][39]

Medacs specifically praised the "exclusive" contract with the DHSC "to support the national Covid-19 testing programme" and the NHS "Vaccination programme" for its significant revenue growth during the pandemic.

Prior to the eye-watering £350 million deal, Medacs had previously worked with numerous councils across England during the pandemic. The public version of the_contract between government and Medacs was heavily redacted prior to publication, resulting in key sections being obscured from public view – including the 'contract charges' and details of the services being provided.

In December 2020, Medacs released a statement saying that it was "delighted" to be working "in building a workforce for the National Vaccination Programme".

Shadow Cabinet Office minister Rachel Reeves told openDemocracy at the time: "People are understandably furious seeing businesses owned and run by the friends and donors of the Tory Party being awarded huge multi-million-pound public contracts throughout this pandemic.

"Cronyism, incompetence and waste have been everyday features of this government's approach to outsourcing and ministers show little willingness to learn lessons from the NAO investigations."

Medacs was criticised pre-pandemic in 2019 when a Care Quality Commission report on a homecare service run by the firm was rated "inadequate".

The regulator found "that the care people received was not

safe. The majority of people's care calls were not delivered at the time they were expected and people gave examples of where this had impacted significantly upon them and the safety of the care that they received."

Furthermore the report noted that "medicines records were not kept up to date and CQC identified instances where medicines records showed a potential overdose".[40]

At the time, Medacs said that the poor rating was down to a lack of staff after the firm won a series of contracts in quick succession. "These award successes were characterised by an unprecedented shortfall in staff transferring from the outgoing providers," the director of the company's Croydon care home said.

"We have invested in new staff and in additional training and support as a priority measure," she added.

Lord Ashcroft is one of the largest Conservative donors on record. In 2010, an Electoral Commission investigation cleared him of any wrongdoing after one of his companies, Bearwood Corporate Services, channelled more than £5m to the Tories.

Ashcroft, who famously fell out with the former Conservative prime minister David Cameron, re-emerged as a party donor in 2017, joining the Leader's Group of top donors. Among his recent donations was £100,000 towards Shaun Bailey's bid to become the next mayor of London.

When I approached the DHCS for comment about the huge contract award to Medacs, a spokesperson for the department said: "As part of our response to this unprecedented global pandemic, we rightly have drawn on the expertise of a number of organisations to support this important work. This includes when establishing the largest diagnostic network in British history, and a test and trace system used by tens of millions of people to reduce rates of Coronavirus. Proper due diligence is carried out on all government contracts."

Ashcroft was awarded a peerage in 2000, 25 years ago. The next case study in this chapter will concentrate on one of the newest members to the House of Lords, former Prime Minister David Cameron, who was elevated to the title of Lord Cameron of Chipping Norton in November 2023, when Rishi Sunak made the surprise decision to appoint Cameron as his new foreign secretary.[41]

Lord Cameron and the Greensill scandal

After stepping down as prime minister in 2016 following the Brexit referendum, David Cameron embarked on a new chapter in his career. He took on a number of new roles in various sectors. One significant venture was his involvement with Greensill Capital, a financial services company, where Cameron served as an advisor – a decision that would soon pave the way for one of the biggest lobbying scandals in recent years.

Lex Greensill is an Australian financier and the founder of Greensill Capital, a now-defunct financial services company specialising in supply chain finance. Greensill grew up on a sugar cane farm in Queensland, Australia, and went on to establish himself as a prominent figure in the world of finance which in turn made him a billionaire.[42]

Greensill Capital, founded in 2011, gained attention for its supply chain financing model, which involved providing working capital to companies by paying their invoices early in exchange for a fee. The company's business model centred around offering short-term credit to suppliers, allowing them to access funds sooner than they would through traditional payment terms.

David Cameron became an advisor to Greensill Capital

in 2018, where he played a role in promoting the company's supply chain finance services. This advisory role involved lobbying government officials on behalf of Greensill Capital and advocating for policies that would benefit the company's business interests. In 2020, during the early stages of the pandemic, Cameron sent a barrage of text messages (62 in total) to the then chancellor, Rishi Sunak, and health secretary Matt Hancock along with a host of senior civil servants.[43][44]

In total Cameron's informal approaches to ministers included the sending of nine WhatsApp messages to Rishi Sunak, 12 messages to the permanent secretary at the Treasury, Sir Tom Scholar, and a further two to Richard Sharp who was an advisor to Sunak at the time.

Cameron also bombarded five other government ministers with messages, emails and phone calls. The ministers in question were Matt Hancock, Michael Gove, Nadhim Zahawi, John Glen and Jesse Norman.

The former PM also sent four emails and a text message to Sir Jon Cunliffe, the deputy governor of the Bank of England, as well as seven messages to Boris Johnson's senior advisor Sheridan Westlake.

In one cosy text message to Sir Tom Scholar on 6 March 2020, when the financial markets were plummeting, Cameron said "I am riding to the rescue with supply chain finance with my new friend Lex Greensill" before criticising the Bank of England's approach to the turmoil in the markets. He signed off the exchange by adding "see you with Rishi's for an elbow bump or foot tap. Love. Dc."[44]

Throughout April 2020, Cameron peppered Michael Gove, Rishi Sunak and Scholar with further messages. A timeline of the exchanges was summarised by the *Guardian* newspaper and copied here as follows:[45]

Cameron text to Gove on 3 April 2020: "I know you are manically busy – and doing a great job, by the way (this is bloody hard and I think the team is coping extremely well). But do you have a moment for a word? I am on this number and v free. All good wishes Dc."

Cameron text message to Rishi Sunak at 19.05 on 3 April 2020: "First thing would be fine – I can imagine how busy you must be. You are doing a great job – keep going! Speak tomorrow. Dc."

Cameron texted Gove again, one minute later, at 19.06: "Ta. Am now speaking to Rishi first thing tomorrow. If I am still stuck, can I call you then? Thanks! Dc."

Cameron sent a follow-up text to Sunak the next day 4 April 2020 at 08.14: "Rishi – ready to speak whenever you are free. Just sent a one pager that I hope clarifies things. Really appreciate your time. Best wishes. Dc."

One hour later, on 4 April 2020 Cameron texted Scholar: "Good chat with CX [the chancellor]. Ultimately my ask was for one more high-level chat – Charles [Roxborough, the second permanent secretary to HM Treasury], you and Lex – to see if these objections about boundaries and precedents can't be overcome. He agreed, We can do that anytime today or tomorrow. Meantime, could you possibly call Lex to get his perspective on how fixable this is? Might make the main conversation much shorter …. I am really grateful. Best, DC."

At 09.39 on the same day, 4 April 2020, Cameron sent another message to Sunak: "Really grateful for your engagement on this… As I said if there is anything else I can help with, just let me know."

The next day, 5 April 2020, Cameron texted Gove again, referring to Sunak. He said: "He's doing a great job. could I call you at 7?"

On 22 April 2020, after the Treasury refused to grant Greensill access to the Covid Corporate Financing Facility (CCFF) emergency loan scheme, Cameron tried again, sending a long three-paragraph text to Sunak: "Apologies for troubling you again, but I can't see the case against helping to fund supply chains and SMEs in this way… Could you try and give it another nudge over the finish line".

At no point during Cameron's lobbying blitz of government ministers and officials did he declare his true financial stake in Greensill or the fact that he was a shareholder. An investigation by BBC's *Panorama* obtained documents that suggest the former prime minister may have made at least £7 million out of his ties with Greensill. This sum included the cashing-in of shares valued at £3.3 million in 2019 on top of a £720,000 salary and a £504,000 bonus. Cameron, who disputed these figures, also enjoyed access to Lex Greensill's private jet, which he used to fly to his holiday home in Cornwall.[46]

On 8 March 2021, despite Cameron's sustained lobbying efforts, Greensill entered into administration, after the Swiss bank Credit Suisse withdrew insurance cover for Greensill amid concerns over the firm's "huge exposure" to the struggling steel giant GFG Alliance controlled by Sanjeev Gupta.[47]

Cameron's direct access to ministers during the pandemic caused huge public outrage and forced the Cabinet Office into launching a review led by corporate lawyer Nigel Boardman into the scandal. The review found that Lex Greensill was afforded "extraordinary privileged" access to No. 10 Downing Street. The report also criticised Cameron for understating the true nature of his relationship to Greensill and found the transparency around corporate lobbying needed to improve, as the current system allowed high-level access to a "privileged few". Boardman also said that Cameron hadn't broken the rules.[48]

Working for Greensill was incredibly lucrative for Cameron; however, the British public hasn't been so lucky. A report published by the House of Commons Treasury Committee in July 2021 and titled 'Lessons from Greensill Capital' discovered the cost to the taxpayer for Greensill going bust could rise to as much as £5 billion.[49]

The report included the following statement from the late Lord Myners, who argued, "The accumulated losses from Greensill for the taxpayer, in my judgement, are going to be north of £1 billion, of which nearly a half will come as a result of the BEIS Department's scheme to accredit Greensill as a lender under the coronavirus loan scheme". However, this figure is contested by the HM Treasury, whose view is that the costs will be much lower.

Myners also provided further narrative on the indirect costs associated with Greensill's collapse: "You have the externalities, the indirect costs, the cost of having to rescue the steel industry from its saviour, Mr Gupta, and the cost of dealing with the social implications of closure of plant, if necessary, or the net present value of up-front subsidies to keep the steel industry in its current form operating. We are going to be talking about a figure, I would have thought, somewhere in the region of £3 billion to £5 billion".

Three years on from the lobbying scandal that rocked Westminster and GFC is still under investigation by the Serious Fraud Office over its financing arrangements with Greensill Capital UK Ltd. Media reports in January 2024 suggested that David Cameron's involvement with Lex Greensill's firm was still an active "matter of interest".

Cameron's lobbying of ministers since leaving office has been prolific. In late 2019 he lobbied health minister Matt Hancock on multiple occasions on behalf of US-based, global genomics company Illumina Inc – the firm subsequently went on to secure a £123 million public-sector contract.

A spokesperson for Matt Hancock said he "had no involvement in the awarding of these contracts and all normal processes were followed".[50]

In February 2022, a briefing paper released to me via a FOI request, prepared by health officials prior to a meeting with Illumina representatives, warned ministers "to be aware" of the "significant recent media and public interest in Illumina's relationship with government, due mainly to David Cameron's role as a paid external advisor to the company", an awareness that had increased due to Cameron's parallel role advising Greensill Capital.

In the early stages of the pandemic Cameron also helped an Old Etonian school friend by connecting him with DHSC advisors. The friend was Hugh Warrender, a businessman who was representing a South Korean Covid testing firm and Cameron kindly introduced him to Lord Feldman, another close friend of the former PM, who was working as an advisor to health ministers during this time.[51]

The House of Lords was able to hold a tight grip on decision makers during the pandemic, using political leverage to their advantage. This book has covered a number of those striking case studies. From Baroness Mone and Lord Chadlington trying to influence ministers responsible for procuring PPE or Lord Markham and Lord Feldman representing private interests in the Covid testing market, this unique moment in our history demonstrated the peers residing in the upper house still wield strong influence over society and the decision makers who govern us all.

Chapter 4

The brokers

One of the biggest scandals and remaining unsolved mysteries associated with government procurement during the pandemic was the impact of intermediaries who deployed their political connections within the Conservative Party to broker huge contracts for clients keen on securing a place on the PPE or Covid testing gravy train.

Conservative peer Baroness Mone and ex-Tory MP Brooks Newmark, who were discussed at length in Chapter 1 are typical case studies of PPE brokers in action – both Mone and Newmark utilised their affiliation to the Conservative Party to gain access to multiple government ministers. In total they had direct access to at least six serving ministers and peers – namely, Michael Gove, Matt Hancock, Lord Agnew, Lord Bethell, Lord Deighton and Liz Truss, according to email correspondence.

Mone and Newmark had access that others could only dream of and exploited it to devastating effect. The contracts awarded to PPE Medpro and Worldlink Resources via the VIP lane totalled £461 million – a direct result of lobbying by the duo.

Neither Mone or Newmark had a track record in supplying PPE to the NHS, but this fact seemed inconsequential to ministers at that time. The companies they represented went on to provide unusable PPE that looks set to cost the taxpayer dearly – goods valued at circa £200–£250 million are likely to be incinerated or destroyed before they got anywhere near an NHS trust hospital.

Despite this unpalatable situation, the PPE deals were very lucrative for the brokers. Mone received a reported £29 million into a trust fund controlled by her and her family and Newmark's company saw a £2 million boost in capital. Newmark's business partner and fellow PPE broker Zoe Ley pocketed a further £23 million out of the government contract with Worldlink Resources.

Unfortunately the Baroness Mone and Newmark examples were not isolated incidents and soon a whole cottage industry of secretive PPE brokers was established.

Samir Jassal and Pharmaceuticals Direct Ltd

Sir Christopher Wormald, the DHSC's permanent secretary, revealed in his witness statement to the Covid Inquiry that he ordered officials to cease procurement of FFP3 face masks on 30 June 2020. Yet mysteriously on 4 July 2020 his department entered into a £102.6 million contract with a company called Pharmaceuticals Direct Limited (PDL) to supply 20 million FFP3s. Remarkably health officials had told alternative suppliers just 48 hours previously that the government was "no longer looking to purchase" FFP3 masks. A peculiar timeline of events.[1][2][3]

By the time the DHSC finally published details of PDL's £102.6 million contract in late March 2021, Good Law Project had already become suspicious of this company's dealings. PDL had already secured a £28.8 million PPE contract six weeks prior to its larger second contract. Rumours of ministerial involvement and political lobbying were voiced, but for weeks, I couldn't find the connections; however, that all changed on 29 March 2021 when the government let its guard down.[4]

When the government places a contract with the private sector to provide goods and services, it has a duty to place a copy of the contract award notice along with a copy of the contract in the public domain. Often large swathes of important information are routinely redacted in the published documents and it's not uncommon for suppliers' contact names and details to be completely obscured from view in this manner.

The UK government publishes its contracts on a government-run website called Contracts Finder. The PDL contract was uploaded in the same manner as most of the other PPE contracts placed during this period – late and heavily redacted. However, officials made a mistake and in an apparent admin error failed to remove the "supplier's contact name" from a spreadsheet that accompanied the contract notice. Trawling through the spreadsheet I noticed the name Samir Jassal.[5]

Samir Jassal wasn't a name I recognised. PDL made no reference to him on the website or on any Companies House filings, but it didn't take long to track him down. Jassal, courtesy of his LinkedIn profile, was a partner in an unnamed "pharmaceutical company", but alarmingly he was also heavily embedded within the Conservative Party.[6]

Jassal, according to his online profile, started his political career as a Conservative Party activist in 2005 by supporting the party in the build-up to the 2006 local elections. He also supported two MPs in the House of Commons during this time.

Fast-forward to 2014: Jassal by now had moved up

the Conservative ranks to become the Tory candidate for the constituency of East Ham – he eventually lost out to long-standing Labour MP, Sir Stephen Timms, who picked up 77.5% of the vote.[7]

During 2014–15, Jassal spent nearly two years working as an advisor inside 10 Downing street on "engagement campaigns" associated with Sikh communities and was also an advisor to former home secretary Priti Patel – a relationship Jassal would later rekindle.

By 2016, Jassal was assisting Zac Goldsmith with his controversial London mayoral campaign (eventually losing to Labour's Sadiq Khan) and in 2017, he was again selected to be a Conservative Party candidate in the upcoming general election, this time for the constituency of Feltham and Heston – only to lose out again to the Labour Party candidate, Seema Malhotra, by significant margins.[8]

Photos published online show Mr Jassal campaigning alongside three former prime ministers – Theresa May, David Cameron and Boris Johnson. Jassal continued to campaign alongside Johnson many months after the PPE contracts were awarded to PDL.[9]

On 20 April 2021, working alongside Phil Kemp at the BBC, the first story on Samir Jassal and PDL was published – it immediately picked up coverage across most national news titles. The government implied Jassal was named in an "admin" error and promptly removed any mention of his name from the published records. Jassal told the BBC he was acting as a "consultant" for PDL.

The strong links between the Tories and PDL's broker Samir Jassal were alarming. Furthermore, the timing of the contract in late July (months past the initial first wave of the pandemic) combined with the fact that both contracts, totalling £131 million, were awarded without any formal competition, raised further questions. In April 2021 Good Law Project instructed its legal team to commence the first steps towards legal action.

The pre-action protocol letter sent by Bindmans LLP to the government's legal department flagged the various concerns that we had encountered with the PDL contract and its broker and asked for documentation that would provide a "a full explanation of the basis for the award of the PDL contract, and the nature and scope of the involvement of Mr Jassal in relation thereto". Good Law Project also requested evidence of the decision-making process leading up to PDL's contract awards.[10]

A few weeks passed and on 22 April 2021 the government responded to Good Law Project's request – the evidence they provided was startling. During this time Good Law Project and I were also leaked further documentation relating to the PDL contracts. The combination of the disclosure from the government's legal department and the leaked information painted a vivid picture of Samir Jassal's effective lobbying activities alongside another middleman that would subsequently drag three senior government ministers into the spotlight.[11]

Evidence of excess profiteering and waste was also made abundantly clear in the disclosure provided.

The documentation trail starts on 29 March 2020. Samir Jassal is CCd into an email by Surbjit Shergill. Shergill is another broker working alongside Jassal and PDL. His email was addressed to Munira Mirza – who at the time was a special advisor to the PM Boris Johnson.

Shergill, who had already spoken to Mirza earlier in the day, was lobbying on behalf of PDL and urged to be put in touch with the "relevant procurement personnel" to assist with the medical equipment PDL were selling. Shergill signed off the email saying they were "keen to support the Party and nation through this turbulent time". Within hours the pair received a response back from senior civil servants.

Not content, Shergill emailed Mirza again the following day – by now officials had dismissed PDL's offer to supply ventilators, but they had shown an interest in the face masks the firm was offering. Shergill again CCd in Jassal in the email and again was applying pressure on behalf of PDL regarding the PPE. He also thanked Mirza for the "assistance" because in his view the PM's advisor had "gone above and beyond for us in this situation" – Mirza replied 11 minutes later thanking Shergill and confirmed she had contacted officials.

Four days after the email exchange between Shergill, Jassal and Mirza, procurement officials reached out directly to Samir Jassal asking what PPE equipment he had available – Jassal responded by introducing the official to Shergill and PDL. Within two weeks, on 19 April 2020, PDL was handed a draft contract from the DHSC to supply PPE valued at £58 million, predominantly to supply KN95 face masks. Unfortunately for PDL and the brokers, the government subsequently withdrew the contract in full.

Jassal and Shergill were not happy with the sudden cancellation of PDL's contract and promptly doubled down on their lobbying efforts. This time the home secretary Priti Patel was in their sights. (As a reminder, Jassal had previously worked for Patel as an advisor.) Jassal called Patel about the cancelled order and this was expeditiously followed up with an email to the minister by Shergill on 1 May 2020.

Shergill opened the exchange by saying: "Many thanks for speaking to Samir and allowing me to contact you with my current issue. I am deeply disappointed to learn that our stock of KN95 masks has now, at this very late stage in the process, been cancelled by the DHSC".

Two days later, on 3 May 2020, Priti Patel wrote an "urgent" letter to cabinet minister Michael Gove on behalf of PDL and the middlemen.

Patel told Gove: "It appears as though the government no longer requires this supply from them. However, they have committed stock and secured supply, exposing them to considerable financial risk and pressures. The late stage in which the government has decided not to use them has caused these problems".

Patel added "I would be most grateful if you could review this matter urgently, ensure direct contact is made with this company over the stock they have secured, ascertain what contractual obligations the government should meet and work with the company to distribute and supply these masks".

Michael Gove passed the punchy letter from Patel across to the health secretary Matt Hancock, who responded on 13 May 2020, following an internal investigation. Hancock confirmed in his letter that the KN95 masks offered by PDL were no longer suitable for use in the NHS; furthermore Hancock added "when the HSE investigated the certification from Mr Shergill's specific offer. Their feedback was that there were problems with all four products offered and that the documentation did not provide evidence to suggest the products met the essential health and safety requirements". Hancock concluded the letter to Patel, by saying that he had asked "the team" to liaise directly with Mr Shergill.

Despite offering four products that all failed the HSE due-diligence checks, The brokers continued to pitch new PPE products to the DHSC – again Priti Patel was on hand to assist.

In an email exchange between Shergill, Jassal and the minister, dated 14 May 2020, Shergill thanked Patel for her "intervention" and confirmed they were "now in discussion to offer another product which may help to mitigate our losses". The product in question was "BY Type IIR" surgical masks.

The middleman pleaded with Patel for further help claiming "in light of our diminished commercial position, I would like to humbly ask for your assistance please". Patel swiftly obliged, passing the request for IIR masks onto procurement officials and ministers. Ten days later PDL secured a contract from the DHSC to supply 60 million IIR surgical masks – a deal worth £28.8 million.

In the space of just 11 days PDL's fortunes changed from complete rejection of their PPE proposals to securing a £28m contract courtesy of assistance from the home secretary and the PM's special advisor along the way.

PDL, Shergill and Jassal's fortunes didn't end there – a far bigger and more lucrative contract was now on the horizon.

On 26 June 2020 Surbjit Shergill submitted a quotation to the DHSC to supply FFP3 masks. The particular masks offered by PDL and Shergill were manufactured by Chinese manufacturer Meixin. Samir Jassal, following a similar pattern to the first contract, followed up Shergill's email with further phone calls and emails.[12]

Within eight days of Jassal and Shergill lobbying officials, PDL were awarded an eye-watering £102.6 million contract to provide 20 million Meixin FFP3 masks. The government agreed to pay PDL £5.13 million upfront.[13]

Incredibly, the government agreed to pay PDL £5.13 per mask. This was vastly overpriced when compared to offers for the same mask from other suppliers. DHSC officials raised concerns over PDL's offer, but these were ignored by the Cabinet Office, who were keen to push through the contract.

On 4 July 2020, the day of the contract award to PDL, a civil servant working for the DHSC told officials working in the Cabinet Office PPE procurement team (called the complex transactions team) that the quote provided by Shergill and Jassal on behalf of PDL was "well above the average we are currently paying of £2.69. Per unit. Even with a 25% tolerance £3.36 per unit this is still way above what we normally pay."[14]

To put these numbers into context, if the government placed the contract with PDL based on a unit price of £2.69 per mask (the price paid to other suppliers) it would have cost £53.8 million to procure the 20 million Meixan FFP3 masks. Instead it pushed ahead with the PDL offer of £5.13 per mask and needlessly overpaid by a margin of £48.8 million.

Remarkably, suppliers offering the same Meixan FFP3 mask offered by PDL and at a much cheaper rate were informed by officials on the 2 July 2020 (two days prior to PDL's contract being awarded) that "as of last night we are no longer looking to purchase" the FFP3s and "DHSC now has sufficient supply arrangements in place to meet requirements over the coming months".

The leaked information provided to Good Law Project was also useful in providing an insight into how lucrative the PPE contracts were for the brokers. Trawling through PDL's company invoices I noticed 11 separate invoices between PDL and a company called Dymon Cap Ltd. The invoices totalled £16.3 million – the owner of Dymon was one Surbjit Shergill. The broker, like Mone, Newmark and Ley discussed earlier, was now a multi-millionaire. Extreme profiteering that one could argue was only made possible by Jassal's political connections to Priti Patel and co.

The owner of Pharmaceuticals Direct Ltd, Bemal Patel, also tucked away huge sums of money following the government PPE deals and in April 2022 went on a lavish spending spree. Mr Patel, who had a previous track record of purchasing and developing property, purchased two huge townhouses in a trendy part of Chelsea and Kensington, spending huge sums on the five-storey mansions. According to records purchased from the Land Registry, Patel purchased the properties via a company he controls called Krrish Longridge Limited which was only incorporated in October 2021, just six months prior to these purchases.

In April 2022, the ORCL opened an investigation into Samir Jassal's lobbying activities. It confirmed Good Law Project's findings that Jassal lobbied the home secretary Priti Patel, and that he had also directly lobbied the secretary for state for health Matt Hancock on six separate occasions, as well as Zac Goldsmith who was also a government minister at the time.

Jassal, who responded to the OCRL investigation via his lawyers Mishcon de Reya also confirmed he had a "consultancy agreement" with Shergill's company Dymon Cap Ltd and he received a percentage of any successful contracts secured by PDL.

Jassal has continued to donate to the Conservative Party. In total he has donated £11,000 to the party, including £7,000 since the lucrative PPE contracts. Jassal is now a serving Tory councillor for Gravesham Borough Council in Kent.[15][16][17]

The government PPE deals were also very profitable for PDL too; profits leaped from £1.6m in the accounting year before the pandemic to £13m in the year end to March 2021 – an eightfold increase.[18]

When Good Law Project broke the story in May 2021, a spokesman for Priti Patel said: "The Home Secretary rightly followed up representations made to her about the vital supply of PPE. During a time of national crisis failure to do so would have been a dereliction of duty. Ministers have no involvement in the procurement process."

PDL made it clear that Mr Shergill was "an independent contractor" engaged "on a wholly contingent, success basis". It said that it had "no contractual or financial relationship with Mr Jassal". It was Shergill who subsequently partnered with Samir Jassal.

The transactions between PDL, Dymon Cap Ltd and Samir Jassal discovered by Good Law Project felt wrong. Why were these middlemen paid huge sums of money – was it for access to their political contacts? Good Law Project suspected so, and in June 2021 it issued a formal complaint to the Serious Fraud Office (SFO). The SFO confirmed they were going to investigate, but at the time of writing this book the agency hasn't yet revealed anything publicly about the case.[19][20]

Within a day or two of Good Law Project issuing its complaint to the SFO, the case took another strange turn. Good Law Project were contacted out of the blue by a representative of a highly controversial corporate spying agency called Black Cube – they were offering to help with our SFO case.

This raised red flags almost immediately. Black Cube were infamous for spying on the victims of Harvey Weinstein among other scandals. They also had a track record of defending clients against SFO investigations and also using undercover operatives to spy on researchers – as was the case in 2016, when the group were caught red-handed spying on researchers working for the University of Toronto who were investigating the Israeli spyware firm NSO group.[21]

We were immediately suspicious. Coincidentally Black Cube were back in the news a few weeks later when the *Guardian* published its huge investigation on the NSO group's mass spyware programme – the software called Pegasus was routinely deployed by corporate clients and dictators around the globe and enabled the phones of political opponents, activists and journalists to be secretly hacked.[22]

Around the same time, the representative from Black Cube reached out to Good Law Project again. We declined to take them up on their offer – I was of the opinion they weren't being honest about their true intentions and found it impossible to believe they would be willing to help Good Law Project. We never did discover who was really behind the stunt, but in light of the depressing news surrounding the Pegasus spyware we took the precautionary step to get all of Good Law Project's phones and laptops checked for any viruses – of which thankfully there were none.

One thing I've learned while investigating Covid procurement cases is that box-fresh companies, which either had little funds in the bank pre-pandemic or simply didn't exist before March 2020, could now regularly afford the most expensive lawyers in London and quite possibly the occasional private investigator (as in the case of Baroness Mone) – all courtesy of the excess profiteering made from PPE and Covid testing contracts.

The political scandal surrounding Priti Patel and Samir Jassal was reignited again in September 2024 – four years after the awarding of the PPE contracts to Pharmaceuticals Direct.

Following the Labour Party's general election victory in July 2024, Rishi Sunak announced he would step down as leader of the Conservative Party, but only after a new candidate had been selected to replace him. One of those candidates was Priti Patel.

Ultimately her bid to replace Sunak failed, but not before she accepted £190,000 in donations to support her campaign to become the party's new leader. Patel's biggest single donation of £70,000 came courtesy of Lubov Chernukhin, the wife of

Russian Vladimir Chernukhin – Vladimir Putin's former deputy finance minister. However, it was the former home secretary's second-biggest contributor – Sunbeam Consulting Ltd – that caught the eye Max Colbert and me at the Good Law Project.

Sunbeam Consulting Ltd was incorporated in March 2022 in Chatham, Kent. The nature of its business according to Companies House records was to provide "management consultancy activities". The latest company accounts published by Sunbeam in April 2024 covering the period up to March 2023 suggest the firm had £63,000 cash in the bank, but just £1,000 in net assets.[23]

Sunbeam Consulting has just one director – Mrs Kiran Jassal, the wife of one Mr Samir Jassal.

Despite declaring just £1,000 in assets in April 2024, Sunbeam Consulting went on to bankroll Priti Patel's leadership campaign to the tune of £31,400. From 1 August 2024 through to 8 September 2024, Kiran Jassal's firm provided Patel with a vehicle and chauffeur valued at £21,400 and on 29 July 2024 handed her £10,000 in cash.[24]

The offices of Priti Patel and Samir Jassal did not respond to Good Law Project's request for comment.

Mustafa Mohammed and Ecolog International

In December 2022, when the government finally released the names of the people behind the Covid testing 'VIP' lane, it was revealed that a company called Ecolog International (UK) was successfully referred onto the high-priority route after being identified by Matt Hancock. The disclosure also revealed that a third party was involved in the process too. Genix Healthcare, controlled by Mustafa Mohammed, had introduced Ecolog to Matt Hancock.[25][26]

A quick scan of the Electoral Commission database revealed that Mohammed had donated £234,000 to the Conservative Party, and his company Genix Healthcare an additional £156,000.[27]

Shortly after the discovery, I decided to issue another FOI request to the DHSC and asked officials to provide me with any correspondence between Mohammed and Hancock. At the end of March 2023, the government replied and provided a cache of emails and WhatsApp messages between the pair.[28]

Mohammed and Hancock first exchanged WhatsApp messages on 11 June 2020. Mohammed opened the exchange by saying "Hope you're well my dear friend" and then proceeded to pitch his proposals to the former health secretary.

Hancock replied early the next morning by both message and email thanking Mohammed before saying, "I have asked my team to look into it and get back to you."

A week later on 18 June 2020, Mohammed messaged again to say "Thank you ever so much for your kind help. I am very much looking forward to seeing you very soon". Within two hours Hancock replied "Excellent".

In September 2020, following Mohammed's lobbying, Hancock's department issued Ecolog with a letter of intent to supply laboratory equipment and PCR testing for Covid-19, but for unknown reasons, the government later decided to cancel the contract. This decision led to a £38.6m settlement fee being paid to Ecolog to cover "mobilisation costs" – a move that was branded a waste of taxpayers' money by an NHS head of procurement.[29][30][31]

Mohammed's access to Hancock was not limited to just the Ecolog deal; the donor also lobbied the minister on behalf of another Covid testing firm – Oxsed.

Oxsed was a "spinout" company from Oxford University,

and would eventually go on to supply tests for Heathrow Airport.[32]

On 4 September 2020, Mohammed again took to WhatsApp to lobby Hancock. He started in the message "My dear friend, hope you are well" before saying, "As you will be aware my dear friend I am involved with Oxsed and have been liaising with [redacted] and [redacted] team who have been extremely helpful". Mohammed went on to ask the minister if he could "please let me know if there is anyone else we should be contacting to speed up the process my dear friend".

Later the same evening Mohammed messaged Hancock again: "Thank you for all your help". Hancock replied the following morning and confirmed he would review Mohammed's pitch.

Mohammed continued to lobby Hancock throughout September and October 2020 on behalf of Oxsed.

Mustafa Mohammed was not the only prominent Conservative Party donor backing Oxsed. The firm also had the support of businessman Mohamed Amersi.

Mohamed Amersi is a controversial figure within Conservative Party circles. It's reported that he has donated in excess of £500,000 to the party and its politicians since 2018. Meeting minutes obtained by Good Law Project revealed that on 6 June 2020, Mohamed Amersi met with Lord Bethell and discussed the Covid test supplied by Oxsed. Amersi also emailed Matt Hancock in September 2020 on behalf of a different Covid testing company. In this email, the Tory donor asked the former secretary of state if he could appoint "a single senior person" to "shepherd this along if it has merit".[33]

In this instance Amersi's and Mohammed's lobbying on behalf of Oxsed failed – the firm, unlike Ecolog, didn't secure a direct government contract. But the high level of access afforded to Amersi and Mohammed is certainly alarming.

Both Mohammed and Amersi said they made no financial gain from the contacts and that they acted purely to help in a time of national crisis.

Andrew Mills and Ayanda Capital

On 26 April 2020, civil servants working inside the government's VIP lane were spooked. They were trying to get a new PPE contract "over the line" but were worried of the consequences should the award fail to materialise. The broker facilitating the deal was politically connected and officials were concerned he would "escalate as high as he can possibly go!!".[34]

Ten days previously, on 16 April 2020, the same civil servant was warned to call the broker urgently to avoid him applying pressure at ministerial level. The email read: "This is likely to get escalated to ministerial level in the next 20 mins or so."[35]

The broker in question was Andrew Mills and three days after officials warned that he would complain to ministers, the firm he was representing landed a £252 million PPE contract to provide face masks. The contract awarded to Ayanda Capital was highly controversial and Mills played a central role in facilitating the deal.[36]

So who is Andrew Mills? He is a UK businessman who prior to the pandemic was a "board advisor" to a number of British companies. He was the founder of a consultancy firm called Prospermill Limited and in March 2020 became a "senior Board Advisor" at Ayanda Capital. Crucially he also spent three years advising Liz Truss as a member of the UK Board of Trade, from October 2017 onwards.[37]

On 11 April 2020, Mills approached officials via his company Prospermill with an offer to supply millions of face masks and was promptly fast-tracked through the high-priority lane courtesy of a referral from a senior civil servant in the Cabinet Office.[38][39]

At this point in time Prospermill was barely a year old, it hadn't filed any company accounts and had no track record in previously supplying PPE to the NHS.[40]

During Good Law Project's preparations for its judicial review that sought to challenge the government's decision to award the £252 million PPE contract to Mills and Ayanda, it was my job to wade through thousands of pages of disclosure about the deal. It quickly became apparent that Mills' political connections back to Liz Truss's UK Board of Trade weighed heavily on the minds of civil servants and certainly influenced decision-making.

One such example is an email sent on 15 April 2020, just four days after Mill's first approached the government. The email between civil servants said: "Could we treat this as a <u>VIP case</u> please. Andrew (the source) was a Board of Trade Advisor (similar to a Non-Exec Director) for DIT. This will be credible and I'd suggest it should be fast-tracked through the system. [41]

Two days later on 17 April 2020, another email between PPE officials read: "Can we expedite this one please? It's a big opportunity – [redacted] masks – and we are close to losing it. Our contact has close ties to DIT so wouldn't be a good outcome".[42]

As negotiations progressed between Mills and the DHSC, it became apparent that Mills' company Prospermill did not have the correct "international banking infrastructure" in place to broker the deal and it was decided the contract would be issued to Ayanda Capital instead – a company Mills had only just begun advising a few weeks previously.[43]

The DHSC entered into a contract with Ayanda on 29

April 2020, the deal was worth £252 million and remarkably the government had agreed to pay the firm a staggering £41.2 million upfront on commencement of the contract. Almost immediately this particular VIP lane contract started to unravel.

On 3 May 2020, officials began to flag issues with the due diligence carried out prior to the Ayanda contract award. The frank exchange was eye opening:

Civil servant 1: "good weekend off?"

Civil servant 2: "frantic. shit hit the fan"

Civil servant 1: "I thought it would be calm this weekend. What happened?"

Civil servant 2: "due diligence hadn't been carried out on Ayanda (RRT) there is a lot of people covering their own arse"[44]

The health officials who participated in the chat were unaware of a due-diligence report completed by the Cabinet Office a day before the contract was issued and which flagged major concerns with Ayanda. The report noted "No financial information available for this supplier due to total exemption accounts filling and so full assessment cannot be made. Rated red as significant assurances required to be able to progress with this supplier and ensure they have ability to deliver." Remarkably the report was not passed on to decision makers…[45]

Problems with due diligence continued into May 2020, when the bank stopped DHSC from paying a number of invoices to PPE suppliers – including Ayanda. The DHSC's head of finance claimed in an email at the time, "Over recent days, and in particular over the last 24 hours, a number of approved payments have been stopped by the bank who believe there is evidence we may be being targeted by fraudsters and that the supplier due diligence processes being operated by the buying team… are not sufficiently robust." The bank eventually released the money to Ayanda.[46]

The problems didn't conclude with the due-diligence reports. It soon became apparent that the FFP2 masks supplied by Ayanda were not fit for purpose. The government had purchased masks that had "eye-loop fastenings" when they should have been "head-loop" fastenings, rendering them unsuitable for NHS staff to use on Covid wards. The waste was staggering – Ayanda had supplied 45 million unusable masks that look set to cost the taxpayer £145 million.[47]

Despite the obvious failures with the contract, Mills and the Ayanda directors made huge profits from the doomed deal. Mills went to some length to try and conceal this fact, by converting his company Prospermill from a limited company to an unlimited one – unlimited companies aren't required to submit and publish company accounts. However, these efforts were fruitless. Richard Brooks, an investigative journalist at *Private Eye* who was also reporting on pandemic contracts for the magazine's fortnightly "profits of doom" segment, had been passed documents that revealed Andrew Mills was paid an astronomical £32.4 million commission for brokering the deal; furthermore Ayanda and its directors Tim Horlick and Nathan Englebrecht pocketed circa £31 million between them.[48]

From start to finish the Ayanda contract was flawed. The extreme profiteering on display was flabbergasting – £63 million profits on a deal that would likely see £145 million worth of PPE destroyed.

It has been over five years since the start of the pandemic and the names of many of the brokers involved in lobbying ministers on behalf of prospective suppliers remain shielded from public view. The data that has been published by the government on

PPE and Test and Trace contracts often deliberately leaves out the names of the intermediaries who played an intrinsic role in forcing the contract into existence – take for example the case of PPE company Euthenia Investments Ltd.

Victoria Aitken and Euthenia Investments

On 13 April 2020, Euthenia Investments Ltd, a London-based "trading firm" secured a £880,000 contract from the DHSC to supply PPE. Euthenia was not your typical healthcare provider and was only incorporated five months prior to the contract award.[49][50][51]

Euthenia found its way onto the VIP lane. Official records claim the Conservative Party minister Lord Agnew was both the "source" of the referral and the "actual" referrer of the firm. However, this isn't entirely true.[52]

Lord Agnew was not in fact the source, which was defined by the DHSC as "the individual or team that identified the organisation". This credit should go to Victoria Aitken, the daughter of the former Conservative Party minister Jonathan Aitken.[53]

Aitken established herself as PPE broker at the onset of the pandemic and bragged about using her "connections" to get Euthenia's offer "fast-tracked".

Good Law Project obtained communications between Aitken and the managing director of Euthenia Investments. LinkedIn messages between the pair reveal Aitken threatened to sue Euthenia over an unpaid commission for securing the PPE contract.

Aitken claimed she had Euthenia's VIP lane deal "fast-tracked" and pushed for the firm to pay a commission on "all the contracts that came via my connections". Aitken contacted Lord Agnew directly to try and broker the PPE deal.

Lawyers representing Aitken said: "our client would find the relevant individuals within the UK government and ascertain what processes would need to be used in order for Euthenia Investments Limited to be properly registered as a supplier of PPE to the UK government. Our client made some enquiries in this regard and eventually made connection with Lord Agnew's office." Interestingly it appears Aitken was able to contact Agnew on his personal email address despite the minister holding both a Cabinet Office email address and a parliamentary email address.

A private secretary of Agnew wrote back to Aitken confirming he would "get our priority team to pick it up and expedite the offer to assure it, etc."

Aitken's effectiveness at securing the PPE contract was disputed by Euthenia; however, what isn't in dispute here is the ease with which Conservative Party-affiliated brokers routinely had access to government ministers via secretive communication channels – often conducted on private email addresses or over WhatsApp messages. Lord Agnew wasn't just targeted by Aitken. We have seen previously in this book that he was also the target of Baroness Mone and ex-Tory MP Brooks Newmark. Let us hope the Covid Inquiry delves into the murky world of brokers and provides the public with much needed transparency and clarity.

Chapter 5

Private health firms and the former PM

The date when the nation entered into its first national lockdown and the British public braced itself for the full impact of the pandemic, 23 March 2020, is etched into our brains. Just 48 hours previously, the government signed off on a mammoth, multi-billion-pound contract between NHS England and the private health industry.

On 21 March 2020, health officials agreed a deal involving the majority of private hospitals in the country. The contract involved the public sector handing over vast sums of cash in return for securing complete access to the private sector's hospital beds, staff and facilities to treat Covid-19 patients and help the NHS cope with the surge in demand created by the pandemic.

The health secretary Matt Hancock announced at the time, "Under the agreement, the independent sector will reallocate practically its entire national hospital capacity en bloc to the NHS. It will be reimbursed, at cost – meaning no profit will be made for doing so. 'Open book' accounting and external auditors will verify the public funds being deployed."[1]

The government block-booked 8,000 hospital beds, 12,000 ventilators, 10,000 nurses, 700 doctors and 8,000 other clinical staff – at face value, the government's decision to take such drastic action, a deal officials labelled "the first of its kind ever", sounded like a sensible plan. The country was facing a new and unprecedented threat from the virus and there was a very real threat the NHS would be overwhelmed. However, like all the other major procurement programmes rolled out during the early stages of the pandemic (PPE, ventilators, Covid testing), the process and outcome weren't quite as straightforward, transparent or effective as claimed by ministers.

In total 27 private providers initially signed up to NHSE's "national agreement", which was initially valued at £1.57 billion and was due to conclude in October 2020. Major players such as Care UK, Circle Health, Spire Healthcare and Ramsay Health were signatories.[2][3]

From the outset concerns were raised about the lack of transparency. The government was refusing to publish the contracts, stonewalling FOI requests for details on how much NHSE was spending block-booking hospital beds in this unprecedented manner and generally being obstructive with requests for information about the capacity being utilised in the private-sector facilities.

When I started to look at this particular contract in early 2021, it soon became apparent that a number of the suppliers had close ties to the government and the Conservative Party. In a joint investigation with Rob Davies at the *Guardian* we discovered the following.[4]

One Healthcare, a recipient of contracts worth £17.7 million was owned by the asset manager Octopus Investments – in 2018, the same firm handed £12,500 to the Conservative Party.

Ramsay Health Care, which operated 34 private UK-based hospitals and treatment centres, secured deals valued at up to £380m. The firm's general counsel previously worked for the DHSC between 2008 and 2013. Ramsay told the *Guardian* "he was not involved in negotiating the contracts but did work on their coordination and legal drafting".

Furthermore, Tory peer and major Conservative Party donor Lord Nash is the ex-chairman and a shareholder in Care UK. Another recipient of the contract was Practice Plus Group, which was owned by the private equity group Bridgepoint, whose advisory board includes the Conservative life peer Stuart Rose and Alan Milburn, the former Labour Health Secretary. [5]

A month after the *Guardian* published its reports, journalists at openDemocracy discovered that the investment firm Bridgemere group, which held a significant stake in Circle Health, a company awarded a £346.6 million contract to provide hospital beds, held a secretive meeting with Matt Hancock in January 2020 to discuss "NHS use of private sector capacity".

However under closer scrutiny from openDemocracy it was discovered that no meeting minutes or agenda were produced for the meeting between Hancock and Bridgemere – a firm that had donated over £1 million to the Conservative Party.

The DHSC also failed to declare that a representative from Toscafund, another major shareholder in Circle, was also in attendance during the January 2020 meetings. Labour MP Margaret Hodge, the former chair of the Public Accounts Committee, told journalists, "These are deeply troubling revelations. No ifs, no buts – secretaries of state should not be having shady meetings with major Tory Party donors."[6]

The Guardian also uncovered evidence that contradicted Matt Hancock's statement that private firms would only be "reimbursed, at cost – meaning no profit will be made" while executing the contract.

Guardian journalist Rob Davies reported: "Accounts for Practice Plus Group, which won £76.3m of work under the contract, raise questions about this assertion. They state that it worked on a 'cost plus' basis, using a 'cost plus pricing formula'."

Whereas company accounts filed by Ramsay Health Care, which landed a £271.1 million deal from the national agreement, said "it worked at cost price plus an extra 8.6% in infrastructure costs". Ramsey told the *Guardian* that it did not profit from the NHSE contract.

Compounded by the lack of transparency and the emerging political connections, unease over the secretive deals was building. My boss at the time, Jo Maugham, the director of Good Law Project, succinctly summarised the growing concern, when he said in May 2021: "Billions of pounds of public money has been handed to private healthcare firms with hardly any transparency – many of which happen to have links to the Conservative Party.

"No one would fault the government for doing what was necessary to increase capacity to ensure people could still get the care they needed at the height of the pandemic, so what is it that government has got to lose from publishing these contract details?"[7]

Around the same period, the Centre for Health and the Public Interest (CHPI), an independent think tank that specialises in health and social care policies, was conducting its investigation into the NHSE's contracts with the private hospitals. Led by researcher Sid Ryan, in September 2021 CHPI published its findings and they were truly remarkable.

A total of 193 private hospitals in England have overnight beds, of which 187 provided data to the CHPI, who promptly discovered only a tiny fraction of Covid-related patients were treated by the private-sector providers. The think tank summarised "on 39% of the days from March 2020 to March 2021 no bed was occupied by a Covid patient, and on 20% more days, only one bed was occupied by a Covid patient. In total, the 187 private hospitals accounted for 0.08% of the national total of 3.6m Covid bed-days".

The CHPI report also found that during the same period of time (March 2020 to March 2021) "NHS-funded elective care carried out in private hospitals fell by 45%, a shortfall of 291,000 procedures, compared with the 12 months before the pandemic. The government had hoped the deal would lead to the private sector increasing the number of NHS-funded treatments freeing up the NHS to tackle the surge in Covid cases."[8]

One important question still remained unanswered: how much money did the government spend block-booking the private hospitals whose facilities only provided 0.08% of Covid patient care?

NHS England, like most other public authorities, is required to regularly publish details of the payments it has made to private providers of goods. Typically each month the authority would publish a spreadsheet detailing every invoice paid where the value exceeded £25,000 alongside the date the payment was made, but in March 2021 when I logged into the NHSE website I was greeted with a 12-month gap in the data available to read. The last transaction declared by NHSE pre-dated the pandemic, meaning it was impossible to see how much money had been paid to the private healthcare firms after March 2020.

On 26 March 2021, I submitted a FOI request to NHSE requesting a copy of the missing data. For three months health officials continued to stonewall my questions, leaving me with no alternative but to complain to the ICO.

On 16 June 2021 I lodged my complaint. It would take another three months for the ICO to free up resources to intervene on the case and on 27 September 2021, I had a breakthrough – the ICO wrote to NHSE and requested they provide a response to me within ten days.

But, still NHSE failed to honour the ICO's request, forcing me to return to the commissioner's office once more and complain again. On 20 October 2021 the ICO issued the health service with a decision notice, a more formal response than its letter sent in the preceding month. On this occasion the NHSE was given a further 35 days to provide the spend data – if it failed to comply with the ICO's latest demands the consequences could have been a lot higher for the authority.

The ICO warned, "Failure to comply may result in the Commissioner making written certification of this fact to the High Court pursuant to section 54 of the FOIA and may be dealt with as a contempt of court."[9]

On 2 November 2021, nine months after I started the investigation, NHS England finally published details of its spending and for the first time the public could see how much money had been funnelled to private health providers during the first year of the pandemic.

The dataset published by NHSE was huge and split across multiple documents. By the time I had combined them all into one spreadsheet it had populated 39,320 rows.

The data revealed that eight private health providers were paid an eye-watering £1.69 billion between April 2020 and March 2021. A reminder that these companies were rewarded vast sums for providing less than 1% of Covid-related healthcare.

The eight firms that received the money were Circle Health,

Spire Healthcare Ltd, Ramsey Health, Nuffield Health, HCA Healthcare UK, Care UK, Aspen Healthcare and Practice Plus – five of these firms had ties back to the government as discussed earlier in the chapter.[10]

On 20 November 2020, in an attempt to increase NHS capacity and manage the backlog of patients, the government again reached out to the private health firms. Health officials had set aside £10 billion to be spent over a four-year period. Sixty-seven private sector firms landed a place on the colossal framework contract – including many of the companies mentioned previously in this chapter.[11]

Despite falling foul of the ICO in 2021, NHS England soon fell back into a familiar pattern of publishing crucial transparency data woefully late. Details of invoices paid during 2022 were not published until September 2023.[12]

The same eight companies received further payments of £500 million from NHSE between April 2021 and June 2023 – Practice Plus Group collected the bulk of the payment with invoices totalling £415 million paid during the period.

On 30 November 2022, representatives of Practice Plus and Care UK met with the secretary of state for health, Steve Barclay, and health minister Lord Markham. The purpose of the meeting was to discuss "the use of the independent sector in elective recovery". My initial attempts to obtain a copy of the meeting minutes and email correspondence associated with the November meeting were sternly blocked by the DHSC, which claimed releasing the documents wasn't in the "public interest", further insisting the information was too sensitive to be released because it related "to the formulation or development of government policy".

I appealed and eventually the government relented and provided the meeting minutes requested. The released documents confirmed that Conservative peer Lord Nash attended the meeting alongside officials from Practice Plus and Care UK. Nash has donated more than £600,000 to the Tories and is the former chairman and a current shareholder in Care UK.[13]

An investigation by the *New Statesman* in February 2024 found that Lord Nash was linked to at least £3.8 billion in government contracts. Using data compiled by the procurement platform Tussell, the *New Statesman* discovered companies linked to the Tory peer had been paid on 180,000 separate occasions in the past eight years.

Nash is a shareholder in Softcat, a firm that was paid £2.97 billion during the period, predominantly for its work with the NHS. Softcat was paid £343 million in 2022 alone. The report estimated the value of Nash's shares in Softcat to be worth circa £88 million. Care UK was paid £731 million over the last eight years.

The Labour MP Margaret Hodge, former chair of the Public Accounts Committee, told the *New Statesman* it was "completely inappropriate that an individual with political power and influence should be placing himself in a position to be accused of a conflict of interest at this scale".[14]

While analysing the spending patterns of the Department of Health and Social Care and NHS England, another name kept appearing in the payment schedules published by the authorities – The Phoenix Partnership (Leeds) Ltd.

Frank Hester and The Phoenix Partnership

Since the start of the pandemic The Phoenix Partnership (TPP) has been regularly paid millions of pounds each month by the DHSC. When I first noticed the payment I was intrigued, but was too busy on other projects to spend any time digging deeper.

However on 28 March 2023, TPP handed the Conservative Party a £145,000 cash donation; this followed a much smaller £11,300 donation on 3 February 2023. Intrigued by the new development, Tim Picton, a colleague at Good Law Project, and I got to work analysing TPP's links to the government.[15]

We found that the DHSC had paid TPP at least £135 million since the early pandemic in April 2020, primarily for services relating to the department's "GP IT Futures framework" agreement – although as of June 2025, the department has not published a copy of the contract.[16]

TPP was founded in 1997 by businessman Frank Hester, a former software architect who worked in the finance sector. The firm provides "healthcare technology" both in the UK and abroad. TPP's Systmone program is widely used across the NHS, and an estimated 2,600 GP practices use their software. According to TTP's website the company currently stores 50 million patient records on its databases. During the pandemic TPP was also drafted in by the NHS to provide support on the Covid vaccination programme.[17][18]

In December 2022, Frank Hester penned an open letter that he subsequently posted on his social media feeds criticising the NHS which in his opinion had wasted "hundreds of millions of pounds from the NHS budget" on overpriced IT systems. Hester wrote, "We are here for our NHS. We are here to help, not drive profits for shareholders or to grease revolving doors. Let's do it for the frontline and choose to digitise in an entirely different way."[19]

Hester's claim that TPP was not driven by profit is rather ironic when you compare his comments alongside the firm's annual returns filed with Companies House and covering the same period.

Hester and his company have made eye-watering profits in recent years, predominantly driven by government contracts. In accounts published on Companies House the firm reported a £90 million operating profit in 2022 and 2023. TPP also paid out £23 million in dividends during the same period to its parent company, which is ultimately owned by Hester. Since 2016, TPP has been paid over £440 million for its public-sector work – predominantly courtesy of the firm's contracts with the NHS and DHSC.[20]

Throughout 2022 and 2023 TPP met with health ministers on at least three occasions. One such meeting was held on 12 July 2022. Transparency data published by the DHSC confirmed the secretary of state Steve Barclay met Hester's firm to discuss "technology and product development in healthcare".[21]

After a six-month FOI battle, I eventually managed to obtain a copy of the emails between TPP and civil servants who were tasked with organising the meeting, along with a copy of the attendance list. However the government refused to provide me with a copy of the meeting minutes or ministerial briefing papers produced prior to the meeting. According to officials it would not be in the "public interest" to release the documents and that publication might "prejudice the commercial interests" of TPP.

Interestingly the attendance list provided by the government confirmed Steve Barclay and Frank Hester were in attendance alongside staff from the DHSC and TPP only – no other officials from across Whitehall were named on the list. However, an email dated 11 July 2022, one day prior to the meeting, contained the subject header "meeting TPP UK and the Prime Minister's Health Advisor". It's unclear from the information provided what role the PM's team played in the meeting – the meeting on 12 July came just five days after

Boris Johnson announced his intentions to step down as prime minister.

A week after the meeting on 19 July 2022, Ashley Brook, a director at TPP, emailed DHSC officials. The message contained four attachments including a briefing on what the government could do to drive "productivity/efficiency gains" inside England's GP practices. Most striking of all, the email revealed that Hester's team wanted to obtain VIP access to health minister Steve Barclay. The email read: "During the meeting, we mentioned that there should be a direct line of communication between the Secretary of State and my CEO Frank Hester if required. If at any point this is needed then Frank is contactable on [redacted] or [redacted]". It's unclear if the DHSC accepted TPP's invitation.

Prior to publishing the report regarding TPP's dealings with the DHSC, I approached Frank Hester and his company for comment and questioned them about the £145,000 donation to the Tories.

On 28 June 2023 a TPP spokesperson replied to my request, and said: "The two donations should have been submitted by Mr Hester in his personal capacity rather than through the business. Mr Hester repaid the company in full after the donations had been made. For absolute clarity, TPP is unequivocally apolitical."

TPP's statement was highly questionable, as of April 2024 the Electoral Commission still listed TPP as the donor and not Hester. And the claim that TPP was "unequivocally apolitical" was blown out of the water in September 2023, when the Tories accepted a £5 million donation from the company. Frank Hester also personally handed a further £5 million to the Conservative Party on 16 May 2023. Suddenly Hester and his company were the Conservative Party's largest ever donors. Hester's newly acquired fame following the £10 million donations quickly caught the eye of journalists at the *Guardian*.[22][23][24]

On 11 March 2024, *Guardian* journalists Rowena Mason, Matthew Weaver and Henry Dyer published a damning report about Frank Hester. The outcome of their investigation dominated the national news cycle for weeks and forced Rishi Sunak into a difficult position over his party's decision to accept £10 million from a man now firmly at the centre of a political storm.

The Guardian had obtained evidence of Hester making racist remarks about Labour MP Diane Abbott during a 2019 meeting held at TPP's headquarters in Leeds. According to reports Hester told colleagues that looking at Abbott made him "want to hate all black women " before claiming the MP "should be shot".[25]

In another exchange published by the *Guardian*, Hester reportedly said "we take the piss out of the fact that all our Chinese girls sit together in the Asian corner".[26]

The newspaper published the full tirade made by Hester which initially took aim at an executive from another organisation. According to the *Guardian*, the TPP boss said: "She's shit. She's the shittest person. Honestly I try not to be sexist but when I meet somebody like [the executive], I just…

"It's like trying not to be racist but you see Diane Abbott on the TV and you're just like, I hate, you just want to hate all black women because she's there, and I don't hate all black women at all, but I think she should be shot.

"[The executive] and Diane Abbott need to be shot. She's stupid… If we can get [the executive] being unprofessional we can get her sacked. It's not as good as her dying. It would be much better if she died. She's consuming resources. She's eating food that other people could eat. You know?"[27]

Hester issued a statement once his racist views were made

public. In it he said: "He rang Diane Abbott twice today to try to apologise directly for the hurt he has caused her, and is deeply sorry for his remarks. He wishes to make it clear that he regards racism as a poison which has no place in public life."

The Labour Party immediately called for the Conservative Party to repay the £10 million donation – a request Rishi Sunak refused to comply with.

Three days later, in an extraordinary twist, Catherine Neilan reporting for the *Tortoise* revealed the Tory Party were sitting on a further, undeclared £5 million donation from Hester – bringing the total amount donated into the Tory war chest to an unprecedented £15 million. [28]

On 18 March 2024, in the wake of Frank Hester's vile remarks about Diane Abbott, the NHS England boss Amanda Pritchard condemned the "racist, sexist and violent" remarks made by the TPP boss and record-breaking Tory donor.

Pritchard said in her weekly "healthcare leaders update" she understood the "shock and disgust" that many NHS staff had experienced after Hester's comments were revealed in the explosive *Guardian* investigation.[29]

However, remarkably on the following day (19 March 2024) the NHS awarded a new contract to the Phoenix Partnership Ltd, a five-year, £4.4 million contract for the provision of a "Child Health Information IT System" in the East Midlands.

Details of the award were first published by the government on 23 April 2024, but the contract was not published alongside the award notice; therefore details of the work being undertaken by Frank Hester's firm remain limited.[30]

Hester's ties to Prime Minister Rishi Sunak appear to have tightened since the mega donations. In early November 2023, Hester attended Sunak's AI summit with Twitter/X owner Elon Musk. Hester posted a picture of himself chatting to

Musk during the event along with the text "was delighted to witness the brilliant AI discussion between @RishiSunak and @elonmusk. Really interesting views and insights. Was great to chat with Elon after the conference too. Exciting times ahead in the world of #AI".[31]

Two weeks after the AI summit on 23 November 2023, Rishi Sunak enjoyed the use of Frank Hester's private helicopter. The PM accepted the perk, valued at £15,900, and used it to travel to a Conservative Party event. Sunak has a taste for travelling to Conservative Party events via VIP transportation. In May 2023 he also accepted a £9,000 ride from a helicopter owned by Steve Parkin – the former owner of Clipper Logistics, a firm that had been paid £170 million by the government to distribute PPE during the pandemic (Clipper's contract award is discussed further in Chapter 6).[32]

Rishi Sunak and the private health giants

When Rishi Sunak seized power of the Conservative Party in 2022, following Liz Truss's calamitous two-month premiership, the former hedge fund manager became the UK's richest ever prime minister. The combined wealth of Sunak and his wife Akshata Murty was estimated at over £500 million. The source of this unimaginable wealth was predominantly via Murty's shareholding in the Indian IT giant Infosys – a company founded by her father, N. R. Narayana Murthy and valued at £52 billion.[33]

Infosys's influence appears to be increasing in the UK. In 2023, payments to the firm from the UK government and other public-sector bodies increased by nearly 50% compared to the previous 12 months as invoices totalling £7 million were paid.[34]

Up to the end of 2022, the government had published details of multiple contracts to Infosys worth a combined total of at least £64 million. The published contracts included a £5.2 million contract award from the Care Quality Commission (CQC) in 2020, a £0.35 million contract from the MHRA in 2023 and a £7.4 million contract from the Home Office in 2017. At least £47 million worth of these contracts have been awarded to Infosys since Rishi Sunak became the chancellor in February 2020.[35][36]

The true figure is likely to be higher due to the NHS not always publishing details of its contracts in the public domain. In April 2023, following a Freedom of Information request, NHS Professionals Ltd, an organisation owned by the Department of Health and Social Care which provides temporary staff to the NHS, confirmed that it had awarded Infosys 11 contracts since the start of the pandemic in 2020 and covering a period up to February 2023. However, none of these contracts have been published on the government's contract portal and to date Infosys have been paid £1.6 million via these awards.

In late 2023, I noticed Infosys had suddenly started picking up new contract awards. Some were not surprising and included an extension to a previously awarded contract from the CQC; however, alongside the relatively low-value awards, Infosys landed itself a place on two huge framework contracts that have the potential to vastly eclipse the amount earned from the previous UK public-sector contracts secured to date.

In October 2023, Infosys was named as a "partner" alongside 61 other firms on the Financial Conduct Authority's (FCA) four-year framework agreement to provide IT services.

The FCA's huge agreement is valued at £562 million and is intended to run from September 2023 to September 2027. Other partners on the framework include Fujitsu, Deloitte and

Tata Consultancy services. The FCA is shrouded in secrecy and a copy of the agreement has not yet been published.[37]

Two months later, the NHS revealed Infosys had been chosen to partner with the health service on a £250 million, two-year-long framework agreement alongside 25 other suppliers. According to the contract notice published online, the services provided under the contract include a "contractual vehicle to support the adoption, implementation and on-going development of Intelligent Automation across Approved Organisations." In a similar fashion to the earlier FCA deal, the NHS had also decided to not disclose a copy of the contract. [38]

Suddenly, the value of UK public-sector contracts and framework agreements awarded to Infosys had leaped from £64 million in 2022 to £878 million by the end of 2023 – albeit unlikely Infosys would secure the full contract value from these huge deals.

2023 was also a good year for Rishi Sunak's wife, Akshata Murty: she received a £13.5 million dividend payment courtesy of her shareholding in Infosys – a sum higher than the salary of every Labour MP combined according to reports at the time. Infosys also reported £600m profits on turnover of £3.6 billion during the same year.[39]

In August 2023, Sunak became embroiled in a conflict of interest row. The UK had begun "intensive talks" with the Indian government over a potential trade deal between the two countries. A key demand from officials in India was to allow more visas for Indian workers in industries such as artificial intelligence and IT – an aspect of the deal that would likely benefit Infosys as it sought to expand in the UK. Critics feared this could also lead to Sunak and Murty personally benefiting from the proposed arrangement.

Sunak was due to fly out to Delhi two weeks later to attend the G20 summit, but also to hold a "bilateral meeting with India's Prime Minister, Narendra Modi". According to a report in the *Guardian*, leading trade experts and MPs said there were "concerns at the highest levels of government", and one expert said the PM should completely recuse himself from the negotiations between the two countries.[40]

Sunak also found himself in trouble again in August after it was revealed that Infosys had signed a $1.5 billion deal with fossil fuel giant BP – two months later Sunak announced plans to open up hundreds of new licences for oil and gas exploration in the North Sea.[41]

A month after the *Guardian*'s report on Sunak's conflicting interests, the government published its latest round of transparency data. As I did my usual trawl through the many datasets published that day I noticed an interesting declaration published by the Department for Business and Trade (DBT) – a meeting involving trade minister Lord Johnson and Infosys. The purpose of the meeting, held on 27 April 2023, was to "discuss operations in the UK".[42]

On 8 November 2023, I submitted a FOI request to the DBT. I asked the department to provide me with a copy of the meeting minutes between Lord Johnson and Infosys along with a copy of the attendance list and any ministerial briefing papers handed to Johnson prior to the meeting.

Like Rishi Sunak, Lord Johnson also had a major conflict of interest. Somerset Capital Management LLP, founded by Lord Johnson and Tory MP Jacob Rees-Mogg, owned a £105m stake in Infosys. Alarmingly, working with Nick Sommerlad at the *Mirror*, we discovered the shareholding was increased by around £18m shortly after Lord Johnson held the April 2023 meeting with Infosys.

Public filings show that Somerset Capital held 6.6 million Infosys shares prior to the April 2023 meeting. By June 2023 this had increased to 7.2 million shares and by September 2023 Somerset increased its holdings further to 7.7 million shares.[43]

The government replied on 30 November 2023 and refused my request. According to officials it was not in the "public interest" to provide me with the meeting minutes. The DBT said: "It is important for the companies that the Department for Business and Trade (DBT) engages with can talk freely and frankly with government and they can expect confidence to be maintained in market-sensitive communications with the Department; disclosure of company discussions could undermine confidence in DBT which would deter companies from engaging with government in future" I appealed the decision later the same day.

Two months later, on 30 January 2024, having considered my appeal the government decided to release the documents to me, albeit heavily redacted. The contents of the disclosure were instantly alarming.

Over the next few days, working alongside Peter Geoghegan and Nick Sommerlad, we dug into the contents of the meeting minutes and ministerial briefing papers and on 3 February 2024 our story splashed the front pages of the *Sunday Mirror* with the headline: "EXCLUSIVE: Top Tory accused of offering 'VIP lane' for Rishi Sunak's wife's firm in the UK".[44]

Remarkably, trade minister Lord Johnson told Infosys during the meeting held in India that he was "keen to see a bigger Infosys presence in the UK and would be happy to do what he could to facilitate that". At the time Infosys was vying for the huge framework contracts discussed above.

The minister also told Infosys's representative, "We value

the relationship with Infosys and will continue to engage at a ministerial level when requested of us." At the meeting, Lord Johnson also discussed the topic of UK visas for its staff and "reassured" them on the UK economy.

We also reported: "Lord Johnson's four-day trip to India cost the Department for Business and Trade £8,167. Infosys was one of ten firms selected for face-to-face time with the peer. During the one-hour meeting at Infosys' HQ in Bengaluru, formerly called Bangalore, Lord Johnson was given a bouquet of flowers, a tour and lunch. He was joined by Daniel Gieve, chief executive of the Office for Investment, which was launched by Mr Sunak when he was Chancellor'.

The backlash from Sunak's opponents was instant. Shadow paymaster general Jonathan Ashworth said: "After the Tories handed billions in taxpayers' cash to cronies for duff PPE, the public will wonder why an outfit so personally close to Rishi Sunak appears to have been granted this VIP access. There are serious questions to answer."

Furthermore the Liberal Democrats' deputy leader Daisy Cooper said: "This government seems intent on wrecking the public's trust in politics. The public has a right to know what the government is up to. We must have full transparency of all government dealings with a firm so closely linked to the Prime Minister."

Sunak's astonishing wealth derived from Murty's shareholding in Infosys is also topped up each year by income he receives from his private investments.

The nature of the investments and the companies Sunak has chosen to invest in remain a closely guarded secret. The list of ministers' interests published by the government provides no meaningful detail and simply states his financial interests are controlled via a "Blind trust / blind management arrangement".[45]

In the years from 2020, when Sunak was appointed chancellor of the exchequer, through to 2023, the PM's income from his secret investments increased consecutively and considerably year on year.

Sunak's combined income from his government salary, private investments and capital gains in 2019/20 totalled £1.01 million; in 2020/21 this increased to £1.77 million. By 2021/22 his annual earnings had leaped to £1.97 million.[46]

By 2022/23, during Sunak's first year as PM, the government revealed his earning skyrocketed again by £250,000 up to £2.2 million. The "tax returns" published by Sunak left one small clue as to the true source of his vast and increasing wealth. Contained in the notes section of the return read the following caveat: "All of your investment income and capital gains relates to a single US-based Investment fund. This is the investment listed as a 'blind management arrangement' on the List of Ministers' Interests."[47]

Intrigued by the revelation that Sunak's wealth was being managed by an unnamed "US-based Investment fund", I submitted a FOI request to the Cabinet Office asking for the name of the US company managing the investment fund.

On 27 April 2023, the Cabinet Office responded to my request. Interestingly officials confirmed they did "hold" the information requested, but were refusing to release the name of the fund on the grounds that "disclosure would constitute an actionable breach of confidence" and could likely "adversely affect" Sunak's "commercial interests".

Furthermore the Cabinet Office claimed "disclosure would be likely to harm the company in question's business reputation and weaken their position in a competitive environment by revealing sensitive information or information that is potentially useful in a negotiating position".

The excuses provided by the Cabinet Office were predictable but didn't stand up to scrutiny. MPs, peers and ministers are required to declare any shareholdings in companies that are valued at over £70,000 or total more than 15% of the company's share capital.

Historically, the requirements for ministers and prime ministers to declare their interests are "stricter" than those imposed on MPs. According to the ministerial code all ministers must ""scrupulously avoid any danger of an action or perceived conflict of interest".[48]

The PM's decision to hide his investments behind a "blind trust" arrangement is a growing trend among his ministerial colleagues. David Cameron and Jeremy Hunt were among ten ministers who made use of blind trusts as of December 2023.

The Cabinet Office argues that blind trusts are a "longstanding mechanism for protecting ministers in the handling of their interests". However, a December 2023 article by the *Guardian* journalist Henry Dyer highlights loopholes that circumvent those protections.

The Guardian report highlights, "There is no formal legal definition of a blind trust or exactly what constitutes a sufficiently independent third party to act as a trustee"; furthermore "ministers are aware of what holdings they have when they are placed in a blind trust, and can give trustees general investment guidance that could lead to few changes in their portfolio."[49]

The FOI response from the government suggests that Sunak knows exactly who is managing his so-called "blind trust". Prior to my leaving Good Law Project to write this book, an appeal was lodged with the ICO over the decision to obscure the identity of the US investment fund – later in the chapter we will return to this subject.

One US investment firm that Sunak is familiar with is

his old employer, Theleme Partners LLP – a hedge fund he co-founded before switching to a career in politics. At the start of the pandemic, in 2020, Sunak directly hired John Sheridan, a partner at Theleme, to advise the Treasury on Covid policies.

Theleme Partners LLP's parent company is based offshore in the Cayman Islands and lists the notorious Ugland House as its address. The small office is the registered home to approximately 40,000 entities. In the past, former US President Barack Obama was highly critical of Ugland House and labelled the building as "the biggest tax scam in the world".

Throughout the pandemic Theleme did remarkably well. Company accounts published on Companies House revealed the firm recorded £109 million in profits during the 12 months up to March 2022 – a £65 million increase on the previous year. [50]

Theleme's success during this period is largely due to its fund being heavily invested in Covid vaccine manufacturers Moderna. At the time of writing, the firm holds 7.35 million shares valued at $730 million in Moderna – a sizeable stake that accounts for 38% of Theleme's total investment portfolio.[51]

Data published by the DHSC in September 2022 confirmed 77 million Moderna doses were "deployed" in the UK. In December 2022, ministers signed a ten-year partnership with Moderna to provide a "vaccine manufacturing centre" to enable the production of 250 million vaccines a year. The government is refusing to declare the value of its contract with Moderna on the grounds that the information is "commercially sensitive".[52][53]

It is not known if the former prime minister retained any ties to Theleme or its investment fund after leaving the firm in 2013. However, in 2020, when it was revealed Theleme was a major shareholder in Moderna, Sunak refused to confirm if he would profit from the surge in the vaccine manufacturer's booming share price.[54]

Due to the weak oversight of blind trusts, the British public may never discover who is paying the former PM millions of pounds in earnings year on year and details of the investments he holds may remain shielded from view indefinitely.

Sunak's personal finances after leaving No. 10

In December 2024, five months after Rishi Sunak lost the election to Kier Starmer's Labour Party, I published a report with *Byline Times* on Mr Sunak's business dealings. The former PM had just placed his ongoing financial interests behind an opaque arrangement designed to hide them from public view.

On 5 November 2024, just days after he stepped down as Conservative leader, Sunak registered a new consultancy company with his wife.

The new firm, called The Office of Akshata Murty and Rishi Sunak, was initially incorporated with Companies House as a limited company operating out of central London.

However, three days after news broke of Sunak's new company, the pair made the decision to re-register the business with Companies House, switching from a limited to an 'unlimited' model.

This may seem like a subtle difference, but it is one which has huge implications for transparency and allows Sunak to avoid publishing annual company accounts – a key document that allows journalists and the public to scrutinise the former PM's earnings and business activity since leaving office.

The re-registration documents were personally signed off by Sunak and Murty on 10 November, with Sunak declaring that he is the chairman of the new secretive enterprise.

Little is known about Sunak's new venture, firstly because the company has no website and secondly because very few details are provided in the register of members' interests that is regularly published by Parliament.

Unsurprisingly the only directors listed for the firm are Rishi Sunak and Akshata Murty. However, while Murty has listed her occupation as a company director, Sunak has described his current occupation as "none" – despite being the current serving member of Parliament for the North Yorkshire constituency of Richmond and Northallerton.

The decision to switch from a limited company to an unlimited company is not standard practice.

Former prime ministers Liz Truss and Boris Johnson both established similar companies upon leaving office, but to date have committed to publishing company accounts.

David Cameron, however, has opted for a similar set-up as the Sunaks and his current company The Office of David Cameron was re-registered as an unlimited company back in 2020.

The lack of transparency around Lord Cameron's financial dealings raised concerns when he was appointed foreign secretary by Sunak in 2023, following his involvement in a major lobbying scandal (see Chapter 3).

Transparency campaigners criticised Sunak's decision to hide his business activities. "Increasingly, Prime Ministers continue to play a role in political life after they step back from the frontbench, and receive an allowance to support these activities," Steve Goodrich, head of research and investigations at Transparency International UK, told *Byline Times*.

"Given the quasi-public function of former Prime Ministerial offices, there is a strong public interest in their finances being open to scrutiny. Structuring this office to allow non-disclosure of the details of the company's annual accounts is bound to raise suspicion that there is something to hide."

Concerns over Rishi Sunak's business dealings do not end with his latest business venture, however.

As I mentioned earlier in this chapter, for nearly two years campaign group Good Law Project has been locked in a battle with the Cabinet Office to publish details of the "blind trust" used by Sunak to manage his financial investments while he worked in government.

Between 2019 and 2023, tax statements published by the government revealed that Sunak declared over £6 million in earnings, via his income, dividends and capital gains.

During this time, Sunak served as the chancellor of the exchequer before replacing Liz Truss as prime minister. Remarkably the public have no idea how Sunak was able to amass this fortune, because details of his investments were shielded from public scrutiny.

Pressured while prime minister to release his tax returns, Sunak eventually released a summarised document, which as I explained above revealed that the majority of his income during this period was paid to him via a "US-based Investment fund".

However, further details of those investments have never been released – a decision that Good Law Project is now challenging.

Sunak's family financial arrangements came under greater scrutiny after it was revealed that his wife had links to companies awarded contracts by his government.

Since April 2023, the Cabinet Office has prevented disclosure of details relating to Sunak's investments, so Good Law Project decided to raise the matter with the Information Commissioner's Office, the watchdog responsible for monitoring compliance with transparency rules.

The ICO has now decided that the government should tell it the name of the "US-based" investment firm that controlled Sunak's portfolio during his time in office, but remarkably Keir's Starmer's government is continuing to block release of this vital information and the Cabinet Office has instead taken the drastic action of taking the ICO to a tribunal in an effort to avoid handing over the details. The case was heard in December 2024 and in March 2025 the courts ruled against the Cabinet Office and ordered the release of the information to the ICO. At the time of writing this book none of the information regarding Sunak's US-based investment fund had yet been released to the public.

A spokesperson for Good Law Project said: "Labour were elected on a manifesto that said restoring public trust in politics 'will require a reset in our public life; a clean-up that ensures the highest standards of integrity and honesty'.

"But in stark contrast, the Cabinet Office's continued refusal to share this information shows an alarming disregard for the principles of honesty and integrity, which Labour was so keen to trumpet.

"This is not just about Rishi Sunak. The outcome of next week's hearing will have much wider implications for what all of us are told about the financial interests of the people running our country – whoever they are."

Rishi Sunak's office was approached for comment but had not responded at the time of writing.[55]

Chapter 6

Up in smoke

Covid-19 swept around the world in early 2020 at a remarkable pace, placing an overwhelming pressure on healthcare services to deal with the rapid increase in patients being admitted to hospital. Governments from across the globe quickly began to realise they needed to purchase or manufacture huge volumes of PPE, Covid tests and ventilators at an unprecedented pace in order to meet demand.

The market for medical goods, predominantly manufactured in China, quickly became overheated as governments and their supply chains competed with one another to buy up available stock. This inevitably caused prices to surge as buyers repeatedly resorted to gazumping other competing nations.

The British government spent £12.6 billion purchasing PPE during this volatile period, alongside an estimated £29.3 billion expenditure on services and equipment to support the Test and Trace programme.[1]

Arguably it's understandable that the government had no choice but to spend an extraordinary sum on boosting PPE stocks and Covid testing supplies; however, upon closer scrutiny it was soon established the government had three obvious failings. Firstly it vastly overpaid for goods, even when you consider the difficult market conditions at the time. Secondly, the government purchased too much PPE; instead of buying four months' supply it procured enough equipment to last five years predominantly at astronomical cost. Thirdly it wasted vast sums on equipment that was subsequently found to be not fit for purpose.

The issue was further exacerbated by a lack of adequate controls in place to avoid fraud and corruption during the multi-billion-pound spending spree.

The PPE mountain

It's unclear why the DHSC abandoned its original intentions to build up a PPE stockpile that would last months and instead push ahead with procuring enough stock to last half a decade. Sir Christopher Wormald, the DHSC's permanent secretary, revealed in his witness statement to the Covid Inquiry that his department appointed consultancy firm McKinsey on 23 March 2020 to "develop a single model for demand" that would enable the government to estimate the volume of PPE required for the NHS and social care setting. The model was completed on 12 April 2020. From mid-May onwards the PPE model was updated daily by officials. The daily updates allowed the department to "produce a 90-day forward projection of supply and demand for different categories of PPE".

In early June 2020 the DHSC introduced another modelling programme called the Sales and Operational Planning (S&OP) process; according to Wormald this new system was able to provide a "comprehensive and robust process for estimating future demand for PPE". The new tool was designed to allow procurement officials to purchase enough PPE to cover a 104-day period.[2]

Both of these systems appear to have failed to prevent the government from vastly over-ordering. Furthermore there is evidence that after Wormald gave the instruction for officials to stop ordering PPE in June 2020, large contracts to supply PPE continued to be awarded. Wormald claims in his witness statement that he ordered officials to cease procurement of FFP3 face masks on the 30 June 2020, yet on 4 July 2020 his department entered into a £102.6 million contract with Pharmaceuticals Direct Ltd to supply 20 million FFP3s. Similarly, two weeks later on 14 July 2020 government entered into a £87.2 million contract with Draeger Safety UK Ltd to supply a further 50 million masks.[3][4]

By 30 March 2022, the NAO had concluded its investigation into PPE contracts. The investigation revealed a huge problem: two years after the pandemic PPE stockpile was purchased, 54% of the equipment remained unused.

The NAO found that out of the 37.9 billion items of PPE ordered, remarkably 5 billion items still hadn't been delivered, 1.4 billion items were being held in storage facilities in China and 14.2 billion items that were delivered to the UK remained unused and were being held in storage facilities – including 5.6 billion items locked away in shipping containers.[5]

The 20.6 billion unused items of PPE came at a scandalous cost to the taxpayer; the DHSC's annual report for 2020/21 revealed £9.9 billion was written off the value of the PPE stock. [6][7]

The department confirmed it had wasted £3.2 billion on procuring PPE that was either "not suitable for any use" or "not suitable for use in the NHS". A further £4.7bn was written off due to the inflated prices paid for unneeded PPE, £750 million was squandered on equipment which will pass its expiry date before being distributed to the NHS and a further write-down of £1.2 billion was also required for goods that still hadn't been delivered by suppliers.

The government had another mammoth scandal looming on the horizon – it needed to find somewhere to store and dispose of the mountain of unused PPE stock and it wasn't long before contracts started to flow towards companies linked to the Conservative Party.

Firms who secured contracts to supply and distribute PPE via the high-priority lane were now going to be rewarded again to store and dispose of the unusable PPE.

Uniserve Limited

By December 2020, six months after the government had stood down its controversial PPE procurement channels, billions of items of PPE remained unused and stored across dozens of warehousing facilities around the country. A report produced by the DHSC on 8 December 2020 and marked "OFFICIAL SENSITIVE" confirmed 17,848 shipping containers loaded with circa one million pallets of PPE remained in the country. The astonishing number of containers arriving into the UK crammed full of unwanted PPE had been steadily rising since October 2020. Felixstowe port was in "chaos" partly due to the estimated 11,000 containers full of PPE blocking the quay – ships unable to unload due to the "serious port congestion" were being redirected to other ports.[8]

Officials were desperate to clear the backlog of containers at Felixstowe and in an eight-week period between October and December 2020 approximately 8,000 shipping containers were removed from the quayside and stored elsewhere. Mountains of multicoloured shipping containers stacked five high began popping up in unusual places – a disused airstrip at Mendlesham Airfield in Suffolk suddenly became home to 1,000 containers of PPE; stacks of PPE-laden containers were also spotted at an empty site near Melton railway station, also in Suffolk; and several thousand containers were moved from Felixstowe port to the port of Ipswich.[9][10]

It was a chaotic situation. There appeared to be no strategy from the government on the next steps – what were they going to do with billions of items of PPE currently stored in 17,848 shipping containers and approximately 50 warehouses? While ministers grappled with the situation the stockpile of excess equipment procured during the pandemic remained in storage, a decision that would eventually lead to a further £1.4 billion of taxpayer money being wasted.

An analysis of historic spending data published quarterly by the DHSC demonstrates the department spent a staggering £1.39 billion on "storage costs" between October 2020 and April 2023. This figure includes the storage of PPE and unused Covid tests and ventilators procured during the pandemic. The biggest benefactor of this expenditure was a company called Uniserve Ltd: the Essex based firm was paid a mind-blowing £543.7 million for storage related costs by the DHSC over the same time period.[11]

Uniserve, owned by 62-year-old Iain Liddell, prides itself on being the "UK's leading logistics & global trade management provider". The firm, which shares an office complex with Conservative Party MP and ex-Cabinet Office minister Julia Lopez, has seen turnover and profits surge during the pandemic, predominantly due to a number of lucrative government contracts which have generated payments of £1.15 billion flowing to Uniserve from the DHSC (up to April 2023).

Uniserve's relationship with the government has been controversial for a number of reasons. Firstly, despite the company having no track record of supplying PPE to the

NHS, it was awarded multiple contracts in 2020 to provide vast quantities of masks, gloves, aprons, face shields and goggles. The contracts valued at £303 million were only made possible after Conservative peer and Cabinet Office minister Lord Agnew referred Uniserve on to the VIP lane. Secondly, It was subsequently discovered that huge volumes of PPE supplied by Uniserve under these deals were not fit for purpose. According to data obtained by Spotlight on Corruption, 182 million items of PPE supplied by Uniserve, totalling £178.5 million, were assigned into the 'do not supply' category.[12][13]

Uniserve was also handed a £572m contract in March 2020 to provide freight services to the DHSC. The deal required the firm to assist the government in delivering PPE located in China and South-East Asia to the UK and included the management of sea freight arriving at Felixstowe – where container storage was causing a major headache for officials due to the sheer volume of PPE ordered by the DHSC.[14]

A spokesperson for Uniserve said they procure products for customers, and had a global network of contacts that specialise in PPE. "We did not actively sell our procurement services to the DHSC, we were asked to help".

Uniserve's preferential treatment via the VIP lane ultimately led to the supply of excessive PPE and later the subsequent storage of said PPE came with huge financial gains for the company. During the reporting period covering the years ending June 2020 to June 2022, the firm declared gross profits of £474.9 million – all despite providing unusable PPE that could eventually cost the taxpayer £178.5m.[15]

Incineration

In October 2022, having spent over £1 billion storing the vast volumes of unusable PPE and enriching a number of VIP firms in the process, ministers finally developed a plan to overcome the problem. Attempts to find a home for the PPE mountain were abandoned and the government's new policy was to destroy the remaining PPE – and quickly.

The chosen method was controversial. The chosen contractor to complete the work was equally as controversial. Government ministers had given up hope on reusing or donating PPE and instead made the decision to start incinerating the unwanted medical equipment. Billions of pounds of taxpayers' money were about to go up in smoke.

Health minister Lord Markham (see Chapter 3) told fellow peers in January 2023: "We have tried to donate as much of it as possible to people who want it, but we have to bite the bullet on the rest and say, 'You know what? It's no longer required so we are disposing of it as rapidly as possible.'"[16]

By 30 June 2023, six months after Lord Markham's comments in Parliament, the government had already incinerated 331,113 pallets of PPE. In total 1.4 billion items of PPE had been burnt to create "energy from waste" and that number looked set to rise.[17]

At this point in time, despite incinerating over a billion items of medical equipment, the government still had a further 1.7 billion items of PPE that hadn't been cleared for use in a health setting; expiry dates had elapsed on an additional 108 million piece of equipment; and shockingly, 568 million items of PPE were stuck on hold due to the manufacturer being accused of "modern day slavery". A farcical state of affairs.

In early December 2023, while scrolling through the hundreds of public-sector contract notices published by the government on its Contracts Finder portal that day (by now an almost daily routine I had developed), I spotted an unusual contract that had been awarded by the DHSC a few months beforehand.[18]

The contract was simply titled "Clipper Award – PPE Disposal". I promptly opened the attachment and was greeted almost immediately by a familiar name, Clipper Logistics plc.

Clipper Logistics was previously paid £170 million by the NHS supply chain and the DHSC to distribute PPE during the pandemic. The government was now intending to pay the same company a further £4.5 million to help incinerate the same PPE that it previously helped to deliver. The contract was awarded to Clipper via an existing framework agreement; by now the government had slowly returned to more common methods of procurement rather than the uncompetitive direct awarding of deals that were overly used throughout 2020 and 2021.[19]

Clipper was contracted by the government to deliver the unused equipment to two incineration facilities managed by Veolia UK and SUEZ recycling and recovery UK – which were each handed a £17.5 million deal by the DHSC to burn through 576 lorry loads of PPE every month.[20]

Staying true to form, the founder of Clipper Logistics, Steve Parkin, had previously donated £730,000 to the Conservative Party. Parkin, who remains a shareholder in the firm, was previously a member of the prime minister's Leaders Group – an exclusive group for Tory donors which offered unrivalled access to the PM and other senior party figures. In March 2024, Parkin attended the Conservative Party's elite Winter Ball – an extravagant event where party donors rub shoulders with government ministers and hold expensive auctions to boost the party coffers. During the March event, one donor bought a signed photo of the cabinet for a reported fee of around £115,000.[21][22][23]

The Labour Party's deputy leader Angela Rayner was furious, telling reporters: "The Tories' conveyor belt of sleaze and incompetence has come full circle. They handed millions to a donor's firm with no experience of delivering PPE, then forked out millions more for the exact same firm to incinerate it.

"Taxpayers' cash is going up in flames as the government's bonfire of useless PPE grows. Ministers must come clean about these grubby deals and explain how a Tory donor's company came to be awarded millions on millions for this fiasco."[24]

In January 2024, GXO, the owner of Clipper, had its contract to deliver PPE waste to incinerators extended by a further 12 months – at a cost to the taxpayer of potentially £9.2 million.[25]

Steve Parkin's access to power was revealed further during a November 2024 interview with the horse racing news website the Owner Breeder. Parkin gleefully told the reporter, "My wealth has given me a bit of power in the right places; I could ring Rishi Sunak up now if I wanted to."[26]

Large contributors to the unusable PPE stored by Uniserve and subsequently destroyed by Clipper Logistics and GXO were the companies who secured huge contracts via the high-priority lane.

VIP lane waste

In February 2022, Spotlight on Corruption discovered a remarkable fact courtesy of an FOI response from the DHSC. They were able to establish 25 out of 50 VIP suppliers had provided PPE that was considered by government ministers as being not fit for purpose.

The stats were alarming: 25 VIP lane firms had supplied 475.5 million items of PPE valued at a cost of £1,014 billion that were classified as 'do not supply' – so 50% of all the companies channelled down the unlawful high-priority route had provided unusable equipment.[27]

Lord Bethell confirmed to Parliament on 15 September 2021 the 'do not supply' stockpile of PPE consisted of 1.9 billion items of stock valued at £2.8 billion. Meaning VIP firms were responsible for over a third (36%) of the wasted, soon-to-be-incinerated PPE.[28][29]

Table 3: 25 VIP lane suppliers who supplied 'do not supply' PPE. Source: Spotlight on Corruption.

High-priority lane (VIP) supplier name	Quantity of PPE (nr)	Total cost (£)
PI4 MEDICAL LTD TA PLATFORM I4	20,789,100	£183,567,753
UNISERVE LTD	182,877,570	£178,588,091
AYANDA CAPITAL LTD	44,553,600	£138,116,160
PPE MEDPRO LTD	25,547,328	£124,670,961
WORLDLINK RESOURCE	11,912,785	£106,023,787
CRISP WEBSITES LTD TA PESTFIX	46,688,900	£84,419,554
NINE UNITED LTD	8,007,560	£69,745,848
SG RECRUITMENT UK LTD	2,360,937	£26,477,555
THE PAPER DRINKING STRAW COMPANY LTD	21,889,430	£24,078,373
EXCALIBUR HEALTH-CARE SERVICES LTD	4,459,300	£20,066,850
TOWER SUPPLIES	2,231,086	£10,633,901
MELLER DESIGNS LTD	552,100	£8,464,466
AIYA TECHNOLOGY	368,650	£8,155,335

UNIVERSAL SOLUTIONS TRADING LTD	83,334,025	£7,500,062
VISAGE LTD	3,325,230	£6,268,406
IDEAL MEDICAL SOLUTIONS LTD	995,660	£4,342,510
UNISPACE GLOBAL HEALTH*	153,560	£3,679,298
HOTEL LOGISTICS LTD	3,024,460	£2,587,235
HEADWIND INDUSTRIAL (CHINA) LTD	1,000,430	£2,501,075
INVISIO LTD	8,383,500	£2,221,628
REHEAR LABS LIMITED	723,675	£1,140,512
PIF LIMITED	228,020	£691,032
MGP ADVISORY LTD	100,000	£600,000
EUTHENIA INVESTMENTS LTD	12,290	£57,120
REGAL POLYTHENE LTD TA REGAL DISPOSABLES	2,011,000	£38,209
Total	475,530,196	£1,014,635,721

The wastage levels on the PPE stockpile were colossal, and poor decisions by ministers have cost taxpayers dearly. £10bn literally up in smoke. Lamentably the excessive wastage wasn't limited to PPE procurement; we saw in Chapter 2 the squandering of billions of pounds within the Test and Trace programme through a combination of faulty equipment, surplus stock and excessive profiteering.

There was another flagship government programme launched in the first few months of the pandemic that was also built off the back of cronyism and resulted in drastic, desperate measures being taken by ministers to reduce the waste bill – I'm talking about the Ventilator Challenge.

The Ventilator Challenge

The urgent, chaotic and wasteful rush by the government to procure PPE in early March 2020 was also replicated in its efforts to purchase mechanical ventilators.

Ventilators are vital machines that help to assist patients who are struggling to breath. Anyone who has seen the 2024 ITV drama *Breathtaking*, based on the book by Dr Rachel Clarke, will have seen how important a ventilator is for treating Covid-19 patients admitted to hospital with the virus.

According to the NAO, at the end of February 2020, it was estimated that the NHS had access to just 7,400 mechanical ventilators. A later stocktake would discover that in fact 9,139 mechanical ventilators were available at this time across the whole of the UK and a further 1,156 it could borrow from the private sector – still woefully short of predicted requirements.

By 12 February 2020 and two weeks after the UK's first official Covid case, government modelling indicated that a 'reasonable worst-case scenario' could see demand for ventilators surge to 59,000 units. By 1 March 2020 estimates leaped to 90,000 units – 82,600 ventilators short when compared to the initial stocktake.

The government had a gargantuan problem on its hands and it desperately needed to procure and manufacture at speed the huge number of additional ventilators required to meet the forecasted demand. The government decided on two procurement processes; firstly, in early March it established buying cells to purchase as many ventilators from overseas as it could get its hands on – mainly from China via intermediaries and distributors (more about this further in the chapter).

Secondly, on 16 March 2020, Prime Minister Boris Johnson issued a plea to UK-based manufacturing companies to design and build up to 30,000 additional ventilators. The same evening the PM spoke "to over sixty of the UK's leading manufacturing businesses and organisations" in a bid to boost the home-grown production of equipment. Johnson never declared the meeting in the ministerial transparency data published for this period, so it's unclear who he spoke to on the call.[30][31]

Following Johnson's 'call to arms' the Ventilator Challenge was soon born. The government drive for additional ventilators would eventually cost the taxpayer £569 million and result in many red flags being raised over cronyism claims, excess profiteering, reputable manufacturers being ignored and high levels of waste – a depressing and familiar pattern which chimed with the regularly occurring scandals surrounding the PPE and Covid testing procurement drive that ran concurrently.[32]

A few lucky companies were able, it seems, to steal a march on their Ventilator Challenge rivals courtesy of support from Boris Johnson. Three days prior to the programme's launch the PM had already "talked to" James Dyson and JCB about the government's manufacturing requirements.

The billionaire James Dyson, founder of Dyson, a company famous for its vacuum cleaners, was a staunch Brexiteer and had previously donated £11,450 to Conservative Party MP Michelle Donelan.[33]

JCB, founded by the Bamford family in 1945, is a multinational company renowned for manufacturing construction equipment. The Bamford family have donated over £10 million to the Conservative Party and pro-Brexit groups since 2002, including £600,000 in donations to Vote Leave Limited – the campaign group headed up by Boris Johnson in the build-up to the UK's referendum on its membership with the European Union.[34]

Since leaving office Johnson continued to be bankrolled by the Bamfords. In July 2022, Lord Anthony Bamford and

Lady Carole Bamford shelled out £23,853 for his wedding celebrations including the hire of the marquee, waiting staff, catering and flowers. Johnson even moved into the Bamfords' £20m Knightsbridge property free of charge – worth £10,000 per month.[35][36]

Both Dyson and JCB have a well-respected track record in manufacturing hoovers and excavators, but they lacked experience in building mechanical ventilators for the NHS. This minor detail didn't stop Boris Johnson reaching out to the pair on 13 March 2020.

In a WhatsApp discussion on ventilators, Boris Johnson told Dominic Cummings and Matt Hancock, "We really need to respond and get our manufacturers going. This is clearly a nightmare for the Italians and it will be the same for us all too soon. Have talked to Dyson and Bamford today but we need an urgent number ten summit and maybe find someone to drive the effort. Matt? Gove?"[37]

During the call, the PM also passed the telephone number of Steve Oldfield, the DHSC's chief commercial officer, on to Dyson and Bamford.

Three minutes after Boris Johnson's WhatsApp message, Dominic Cummings promptly applied pressure on senior civil servants by adding, "Who is coordinating the effort with Dyson et al to build a crash programme for more respirators? This is incredibly urgent".[38]

Within a few hours Steve Oldfield had spoken to both Dyson and JCB representatives and the Cabinet Office commenced its contract with Dyson and the firm's designer for the project TTP plc on the same day. JCB was to be subsequently subcontracted to provide the ventilator casings to Dyson.[39][40]

By 26 March 2020, Dyson received an order to provide 10,000 of its newly designed CoVent hospital ventilators from the UK government; reports suggest this order was "subject to the device passing stringent medical tests".[41]

By 24 April 2020, things started to unravel for Dyson and JCB and the government cancelled the contract "due to reduced demand". James Dyson told the press he didn't "regret" the decision to participate in the challenge and claimed "we have spent around £20m on this project to date, but we will not accept any public money".[42][43]

Dyson didn't receive any public money; however, on 15 April 2020 the Cabinet Office paid TTP plc (Dyson's partner in the challenge) £4.44 million despite zero ventilators being provided to the NHS.[44]

A month later in May 2020, the government spent a further £1.2m with a company called Same Day plc, which they instructed to collect and destroy unwanted ventilators and parts including Dyson's CoVent machines deemed no longer required.[45]

The relationship between James Dyson and Boris Johnson made national news again a year later, in April 2021, when it was revealed Boris Johnson and James Dyson were sending text messages to each other throughout March 2020. Dyson and Boris Johnson were in conversation on how to "fix" a tax issue should his staff return to the UK to manufacture ventilators. Johnson signed off the exchange in his usual cavalier fashion by saying, "James I am first lord of the Treasury and you can take it that we are backing you to do what you need".[46]

Leader of the opposition at the time Keir Starmer was not impressed with Boris Johnson's latest cronyism scandal. During Prime Minister's Questions on 21 April 2021, Starmer said "Every day there are new allegations about this Conservative Government: dodgy PPE deals; tax breaks for their mates; the Health Secretary owns shares in a company delivering NHS services", adding "Sleaze, sleaze, sleaze, and it's all on his watch".

Dyson said It was "absurd to suggest that the urgent correspondence was anything other than seeking compliance with rules" and that his company did not receive "any benefit from the project".

Johnson continued to defend the government's procurement decisions made under his watch, but serious questions remain – how were Dyson and Co able commence with a contract to supply ventilators within 24 hours of speaking to the PM and despite having no experience manufacturing ventilators – and all the while companies with a track record in supplying medical equipment to the NHS were repeatedly ignored by Cabinet Office officials?[47][48]

In March 2025, evidence published by the Covid Inquiry would shed vital new light on this contract.

For four weeks, the Covid Inquiry held public hearings discussing procurement decisions during the pandemic. The first witness to be called before the inquiry, chaired by Baroness Heather Hallet, was independent procurement expert Professor Dr Albert Sanchez-Graells. The professor's findings provided further clarity on the political pressure piled on civil servants during this period.

The contents of Professor Sanchez-Graells' expert report were subsequently published by the inquiry and for the first time reveal the true extent of Conservative Party grandee and former Cabinet Office minister Michael Gove's role in ensuring Dyson was awarded a contract to provide 10,000 ventilators as part of the Ventilator Challenge.

Professor Sanchez-Graells' report highlighted one contract included in the Ventilator Challenge – the deal awarded to Dyson in March 2020. The report reveals notably that "Dyson benefitted from preferential treatment" because Michael Gove, the former Chancellor of the Duchy of Lancaster, issued "an instruction" to place an order for 10,000 ventilators from Dyson in March 2020. According to the government's chief commercial officer, Mr Gove was "insistent that an order be placed".

Sanchez-Graells also noted the former prime minister Boris Johnson had "given direct contact details of a civil servant involved in initial discussions to Sir James Dyson".

Furthermore, cabinet minister Lord Agnew also intervened in April 2020 and said: "We are going to have to handle Dyson carefully. I accept that contractually, we can walk away as he hasn't delivered by the due date. I also accept that we have an indemnity battle ahead. But just killing off his design (assuming it gets through MHRA) won't be an option. I suspect we'll have to buy a few machines, get them into hospitals so that he can then market internationally, being able to say they are being used in UK hospitals" before ending the message by stating "Remember he got a personal call from the PM. This can't be ignored".

Professor Sanchez-Graells suggested the Dyson deal could be an "affront" to proper procurement rules and flagged concerns over the legality of the Dyson deal, concluding:

"Favouring Dyson due to the political pressure Ministers were under would have been clearly problematic and, in my view, beyond being objectionable, it would have raised serious questions as to its legality. It would also have raised questions on the origin of the political pressure".

The Cabinet Office, in response to a report on procurement by the National Audit Office, claimed in a press release in November 2020 that "they [NAO] found no evidence ministers were involved in procurement decisions". This claim was repeated on numerous occasions by the former government. We now know this wasn't true.

Ultimately, the initial contract awarded to Dyson was cancelled. A Dyson spokesperson said, "Sir James Dyson responded to a personal call from the prime minister of the United Kingdom, to develop and make a medical-grade ventilator in 30 days during the national emergency.

"Dyson had no intention of manufacturing ventilators for profit. Far from receiving any commercial benefit, there was significant commercial cost to Dyson, which diverted 450 engineers away from commercial projects."[49]

It's worth noting that the government only published the contract between the Cabinet Office and TTP in March 2023, and only after Good Law Project threatened to sue the government over its three-year delay in publishing the required details. Remarkably the Cabinet Office had failed to publish nearly all of the Ventilator Challenge contracts – valued at £248m. Under pressure from Good Law Project the government apologised for the "regrettable oversight".[50]

The £4.4m paid to TTP was typical of the waste incurred on the ventilator challenge. The NAO concluded in its September 2020 report that £113 million was lost on "design costs, components and factory capacity for ventilators it did not buy because the design was not viable or not needed to meet the government's targets".[51]

By September 2020, the government had spent £569m on its ventilator programme, purchasing 20,900 new machines – remarkably only 2,150 had been used due to a lack in demand, resulting in 90% of the new ventilators never leaving the Ministry of Defence warehouse where they were stored.[52]

Three years then passed, with most of the ventilators remaining in storage, wrapped in the packaging they were initially delivered in back in 2020.

By December 2023 the government had decided it no longer

wanted to pay the storage costs and made the controversial decision to start offloading the remaining ventilators. The DHSC's master plan included sending 3,068 machines out to auction over the course of four months between December 2023 and March 2024 – a calamitous decision that increased the wastage bill by a further £135 million.[53]

The auctions

On 15 December 2023, the DHSC signed a £300,000 contract with logistics contractor Kuenhe and Nagel for "storage, handling and auctioning services". The firm was instructed by the government to help facilitate the auctioning of a large stock of unwanted medical supplies, including 3,068 unused Aeonmed VG-70 ventilators. Following the contract award, Kuenhe and Nagel delivered the VG-70 ventilators to British Medical Auctions, which promptly established a number of quickfire sales online.

In January 2024, I unearthed a copy of the contract between the DHSC and the auctioneers and I promptly set up an online account with the auction house. Within a few minutes of logging in, I was greeted with hundreds of lots, inviting me to bid on the VG-70 ventilators. As I scrolled through the multiple pages filled with the taxpayer-funded machines one thing leaped out from the screen – the asking price: £100 per ventilator. A truly depressing sight.[54]

By now I had also established the identity of the company that had initially supplied the soon-to-be-auctioned ventilators – it was a company called Excalibur Healthcare.

In April 2020, Excalibur secured a contract from the DHSC to supply 2,700 VG-70 ventilators. The contract was worth £135 million to the London-based firm.[55]

According to the NAO, the government paid Excalibur

£50,000 per unit. This was a sum that included "transport from China"; however, the NAO said this was "nevertheless much higher than the earlier prices for the same machine" which ranged from £9,000 to £19,000 each.[56]

For every Excalibur VG-70 ventilator sold at auction for the bid price of £100 the government was writing off £49,900 – a waste bill that could top £135 million when the £300,000 paid to the Kuenhe and Nagel is factored in.

On 8 April 2020, two days after Excalibur landed its £135 million ventilator contract, the firm subsequently secured a £25 million PPE contract to supply face masks, The award was courtesy of former secretary of state Matt Hancock who referred the company on to the VIP lane. £20 million of goods supplied by Excalibur under the contract were designated as "do not supply" and were likely destroyed or sold off in a similar fashion to the firm's ventilators.[57][58][59]

This story was infuriating, but did create a positive backlash. Following my reporting with Nick Sommerlad at the *Mirror*, the general public started to donate to a charity called Medi Tech Trust, who were desperately trying to purchase the unused ventilators from the auction sites and subsequently deliver them to hospitals in Africa. My old employer Good Law Project donated £5,000 and the charity also crowdsourced a further £4,906 – enabling them to snap up the unwanted ventilators and distribute them into front-line settings.[60]

The true scale of the wastage on the ventilator programme is staggering. The government spent £569 million overall and at least £248 million has been written off (so far) either in design fee costs for ventilators that were never built or the auctioning off of surplus stock at knockdown prices.

£15 billion wasted on medical equipment during the pandemic

DHSC's annual report for 2020/21 revealed £9.9 billion was written off the value of the PPE stock. The department confirmed it had wasted £3.2 billion on procuring PPE that was either "not suitable for any use" or "not suitable for use in the NHS". A further £4.7 billion was written off due to the inflated prices paid for unneeded PPE, £750 million was squandered on equipment which would pass its expiry date before being distributed to the NHS and a further write-down of £1.2 billion was also required for goods that still hadn't been delivered by suppliers.

By the end of 2022, the DHSC revised its figure and the write-off on medical equipment surged from £9.9 billion to £15 billion – an increase of £6 billion in 12 months.

The £6 billion was attributed to a further £3.5 billion write-down on medication, vaccines and PPE. A *further* £2.5bn was written off the value of the existing stockpile of PPE – a sum according to the Labour Party that would be "enough to fund the police force for an entire year".[61][62]

Not only did the government procurement drive lead to astronomical waste it also created the perfect environment for cronyism and corruption to thrive.

Transparency International define corruption as "the abuse of entrusted power for private gain". They argue corruption "erodes trust, weakens democracy" and "further exacerbates inequality". An example of corruption in the UK could typically be "politicians misusing public money" by awarding contracts to "sponsors".

The introduction of not one but two VIP lanes and the endless stream of contracts and public-sector appointments linked to Conservative Party donors or 'sponsors' one could argue must be called out for what it is – corruption.

In April 2021, Transparency International identified 73 PPE contracts valued at £3.7 billion (20% of contracts placed during the pandemic) which raised "one or more red flags for possible corruption". Their report 'Track and Trace' was an indictment of the government's substandard performance. Table 4 below provides a copy of the report's key findings.[63]

Table 4: Transparency International, 2021 report 'Track and Trace'
– key findings:

High-risk contracts	Twenty-four PPE contracts worth £1.6 billion were awarded to those with known political connections to Conservative Party.
Contracts awarded to companies with no track record of supplying goods or services	14 companies incorporated in 2020 received contracts worth more than £620 million, of which 13 contracts totalling £255 million went to ten firms that were less than 60 days old.
Late publication of contracts	72% (711) of Covid-related contracts awarded during our sample period, worth £13.3 billion, were reported after the 30-day legal deadline, with £7.4 billion of this total reported more than 100 days after the contract was awarded. In comparison, on average it took Ukraine less than a day to publish information on 103,263 Covid-19 contracts after their award during the same period.

Conservative Party ministers created procurement channels that favoured and fast-tracked companies with political connections. These companies were prioritised for contracts to supply, deliver, store and eventually destroy billions of pounds of equipment and all facilitated within the confines of a secretive and unlawful VIP lane overseen by Conservative Party ministers.

Five years later and the PPE waste scandal continues

As the procurement scandal rumbles into its fifth year, it shows no sign of ending. In November 2024 health ministers revealed that over one million pallets laden with unusable Covid protective equipment had so far been destroyed by the government.

In response to a parliamentary question from former Reform MP Rupert Lowe, health minister Karin Smith confirmed: "As of the end of September 2024, approximately 1,049,700 pallets, or 23%, of personal protective equipment (PPE) has been recycled through energy from waste and recycling. The original cost to purchase was £8.644 billion, and all stock categorised as excess has no residual market value."

The purchase price of the unused PPE that has now been destroyed to date sits at £8.6 billion. In total the Department of Health and Social Care has written off nearly £14.9 billion spent on unusable medical goods it procured during the pandemic.

The scale of the waste is staggering. If you were to line up the 1,049,700 pallets of PPE that have been destroyed to date it would stretch for 780 miles – for comparison the distance between London and John o' Groats in Scotland is 692 miles. [64]

The one million pallets destroyed to date is infuriating; however, the situation looks set to get worse. In November 2024, in a Freedom of Information response to me, the NHS supply chain team at Supply Chain Coordination Ltd (SCCL) confirmed that remarkably they still held 506 shipping containers full of unused PPE procured during the pandemic – PPE that was likely to be incinerated or recycled. Incredibly seven of these huge containers had never been opened or inspected – nearly five years after being purchased.[65]

Remarkably, the UK government had destroyed 51,151 pallets of PPE without keeping a log of the name of the original supplier. In a January 2025 Freedom of Information request response, SCCL confirmed the supplier name is currently "unknown".[66]

Full Support Healthcare's billion-pound contract

Full Support Healthcare (FSH), established in 2002, was an established supplier to the NHS for circa 18 years pre-pandemic; it was not a beneficiary of the VIP lane. Instead it was an existing "framework provider" which had supplied PPE during previous pandemics including the Ebola and swine flu outbreaks a few years earlier – so it was no surprise that it should be awarded a contract to provide PPE in 2020.

FSH quickly became the UK's biggest supplier of PPE to the UK government. A BBC investigation found that it delivered circa £1.4 billion worth of masks, goggles and aprons which at the point of delivery were "fully compliant and delivered in good order".

However, the BBC reported, upon delivery the goods were left unopened in shipping containers for several months and may have become "spoiled" after being stored inappropriately for long periods of time – a critique the DHSC rejected.

About 1.57 billion items of PPE were destroyed or written off from this one contract which has now been branded the most wasteful government deal of the pandemic.

Despite the PPE being manufactured to the proper standard, officials have confirmed some 749 million items have already been incinerated, and a further 825 million were earmarked for further incineration or recycling.[67]

SCCL confirmed in a recent FoI request that at least

185,818 pallets of PPE supplied by FSH have now been disposed of. Waste on an astronomical scale.[68]

The government also auctioned off 1,550 pallets of the FSH PPE stockpile and in April 2023 these pallets found themselves crudely stored a farm near a Hampshire nature reserve after they were purchased by another company – Polystar Plastics.[69]

Images of the PPE-laden pallets quickly spread around social media and via national news outlets, prompting an intervention from the Environment Agency, which ordered Polystar to remove the pallets from the farm where they were being temporarily stored.

I approached Polystar Plastics in late 2024 to ask them where they moved the pallets to, but the firm has repeatedly stonewalled my questions.

In March 2024, a warehouse owned by Polystar Plastics dramatically went up in flames. The huge fire destroyed the building and took 100 firefighters to get the blaze under control. News footage captured images of huge flames billowing out from the roof which was only a stone's throw away from Southampton Football Club's sports stadium.[70]

The fire was not considered suspicious by the Hampshire Fire Service.

Documents I obtained via Freedom of Information request from Hampshire Fire Service revealed that the destroyed warehouse was used for the "storage of PPE for the NHS".[71]

Polystar Plastic has refused to confirm if the PPE destroyed in the fire is the same as the pallets of PPE the Environment Agency ordered the firm to remove from the nearby farm.

Wes Streeting, the shadow health secretary at the time, when asked about the Full Support Healthcare contract, said to the BBC the money lost "could have been used to pay the salaries of 37,000 nurses".

"We all know that billions of pounds was wasted during the pandemic on corruption and incompetence, but what the BBC has uncovered is the worst example I have ever seen – £1.4bn on one contract, paying for PPE that was never used.

"It is staggering waste and I think we need a full and frank account as to how so much public money was thrown down the toilet," he said.[72]

The ongoing Covid Inquiry recently started to turn its attention to the procurement of PPE during the pandemic. Live hearings were scheduled for March 2025.

Again, let's hope the inquiry led by Baroness Hallett can force some accountability and transparency over the decisions that resulted in £8.6 billion worth of PPE literally going up in smoke.

Chapter 7

Held to account?

The Covid Inquiry

Public hearings began at the UK Covid-19 inquiry in June 2023 – an independent public inquiry chaired by Dame Heather Hallett established to investigate the government's response and handling of the pandemic. The inquiry has been split into ten modules covering preparedness, decision making and political governance as well as vaccines, procurement, the care sector, children and young people, economic response, impact on society and the Test and Trace programme.[1]

Module 5 of the inquiry covers procurement during the pandemic. This stage commenced with its evidence gathering in October 2023 and four weeks of public hearings were held in March and April 2025.[2]

The scope of the Inquiry's judge-led investigations will consider and subsequently make recommendations regarding the procurement of PPE, ventilators and other "key healthcare related equipment"; importantly it will also review the "high-priority lane". A later module will tackle the NHS Test and Trace programme. According to scope published by the inquiry the following areas will be reviewed during the process:[3]

+ 1. The existence and effectiveness of processes, procedures and/or contractual provisions in place for the procurement and distribution of key healthcare equipment and supplies to the end user prior to and during the pandemic, the suitability and resilience of the supply chains and what, if any, changes were made to procurement processes during the pandemic and have been made subsequently. This will include examination of:
  + a. The overall value of the contracts awarded;
  + b. Preparedness, including pre-existing stockpiles, inventory management and
  + Suitability;
  + c. Spending controls;
  + d. Steps taken to eliminate fraud and the prevalence of fraud;
  + e. Conflicts of interest;
  + f. Contractual performance by suppliers and manufacturers;
  + g. Compliance with public law procurement principles and regulations;
  + h. Openness and fairness, including the 'high priority lane';
  + i. Decisions as to what to buy at what cost and disposal strategies;
  + j. The existence of any maladministration.
+ 2. Procurement of key healthcare equipment and supplies to the end user in the period leading up to and during the pandemic. This will include the existence and effectiveness of procedures, processes and communication between

the relevant bodies of the four nations in relation to procurement and the use made of mutual aid arrangements during the pandemic.

+ 3. The operation and effectiveness of any regulatory regimes and/or oversight (either by the procuring authority or end user) in relation to key medical equipment or supplies during the pandemic including:

> + a. Guidance issued by the relevant advisers, regulators and/or Government;
> + b. The need for, and the efficacy of standards required by the MHRA and the BSI;
> + c. The impact of any changes to the volume, technical specifications and/or quality of the products that were procured;
> + d. The validation process including benchmarks and revalidation;
> + e. Safety concerns (the existence of such concerns and how they were addressed by those responsible for procurement).

As of early 2025, the inquiry has already put a number of senior government ministers, PMs both current and former and advisors under its spotlight, including Rishi Sunak, Boris Johnson, Dominic Cummings and Matt Hancock – at times exposing the true shambolic and chaotic nature of governance inside Whitehall and No. 10 during the early stages of the pandemic. One waits with bated breath to see what the inquiry unearths about procurement and the VIP lane.

The inquiry will not publish its recommendations until 2026 at the earliest, but in the meantime the public has been provided with a snapshot inside government during the chaotic, early months of the pandemic, thanks to the testimonies of civil servants, procurement experts and ministers who were called to testify in March 2025.

During this period I was glued to YouTube watching the live stream from the inquiry as Matt Hancock, Michael Gove, Lord Feldman and co were questioned on their involvement in procurement decisions.

In late 2024, in the build-up to the Module 5 public hearings, I was also hired as an advisor to the UK Anti-Corruption Coalition (UKACC) who are core participants in the Covid Inquiry and as such are allowed to submit evidence, review evidence and attend the inquiry.

UKACC are a collection of NGOs which include Transparency International, Spotlight on Corruption and the Open Contracting Partnership, as well as host of other charities and affiliates. The purpose of UKACC is to "fight corruption in the UK and we fight the UK's role in facilitating corruption abroad" and to "advocate to policymakers, hold those with power to account, and work towards driving real world change" – a fitting brief considering the shambolic decision-making during the pandemic and the unlawful nature of the procurement decisions taken by ministers.

My brief from UKACC was to provide input on its submission to the Covid Inquiry regarding the various VIP lanes (explored in the previous chapters of this book), to review evidence provided by the government and to suggest new lines of inquiry that its lawyers may want to pursue. I also reported regularly for *Byline Times* throughout the months of March and April 2025 – one of the only news outlets still proactively engaged in investigating the scandal.

It became apparent quite quickly during the Module 5 hearings that the inquiry was not going to call in the individual companies in for interrogation, instead passing this buck on to the newly appointed government 'Covid Corruption Commissioner'. Although the inquiry discussed the VIP PPE contracts awarded to the likes of PPE Medpro, Meller Designs and SG recruitment with civil servants and ministers it made the strange decision to decline the opportunity to hear directly from the horse's mouth – not a single PPE supplier spoke at the public hearings. In my opinion, this was a huge and obvious opportunity missed by Lady Hallett's team of lawyers.

Despite this oversight, important evidence did eventually see the light of day and I have included a number of those key *Byline Times* reports below:

The sheer scale of the COVID 'VIP Lane' PPE scandal has still not been revealed five years on – published 16 April 2025

New evidence published by the Covid Inquiry suggests that at least 20 more politically connected suppliers received contracts worth £1 billion.

The Covid Inquiry just completed four weeks of hearings centred on the controversial procurement decisions made by Boris Johnson's government during the pandemic.

Of particular interest was the use of a VIP lane by the Cabinet Office and Department for Health and Social Care to procure PPE – a system that fast-tracked offers from politically connected companies, many of whom had never previously supplied PPE to the NHS.

The previous Conservative government was forced by Good Law Project (GLP) to reveal the names of the suppliers who benefited from the VIP Lane, and in November 2021, finally published the list of 51 names following a long-running battle.

However, those 51 suppliers declared by the DHSC may just be the tip of the iceberg.

In February 2022, Good Law Project was leaked internal DHSC documents that suggested a further 18 companies benefited from the VIP Lane, but this was dismissed by the DHSC which claimed: "It is inaccurate to claim that all of these companies were referred to by the High Priority Lane route."

But, new evidence published by the Covid Inquiry and analysed by the UK Anti-Corruption Coalition (UKACC) now supports the initial claims made by GLP and in fact goes one step further to reveal the names of at least "20 other suppliers who received 48 contracts worth £1 billion" via the VIP route.

Gavin Hayman, executive director of open contracting partnerships and co-chair of the UKACC told the inquiry that "we are still not sure we have got to the bottom of all those VIP contracts".

He added: "It appears that the evidence to the Inquiry on VIP Lane suppliers from DHSC conflicts with that of the Cabinet Office.

"The Cabinet Office evidence appears to omit 20 other suppliers who received 48 contracts worth £1 billion according to the DHSC evidence. I am not sure who is right but it is bad that we still don't know for sure five years on. Hopefully, My Lady, you will get to the bottom of it."

The contradictory evidence provided by the Cabinet Office and referred to by the UKACC is in the form of a detailed spreadsheet now made public by the inquiry for the first time.

But the confusion doesn't end there...

To date, the names of 51 VIP lane suppliers have been made public by the DHSC. However, earlier in the month, the government's former chief commercial officer Gareth Rhys Williams confirmed to the inquiry that yet another company had mistakenly been missed off the list.

That company was Luxe Lifestyle, a previous investigation

by Good Law Project revealed that Luxe were awarded a £20 million PPE deal following an intervention by former Conservative Party ministers and chairman Greg Hands.

Rhys Williams said in his witness statement to the inquiry: "A further HPL company, Luxe Lifestyle, was identified in May 2024 following a review of evidence in preparation for this Inquiry."

Last week it was reported the HMRC were currently investigating Luxe Lifestyle, which led to the arrest of the firm's director, Karen Brost, on "suspicion of fraud by failing to disclose information, conspiracy to cheat the public revenue and fraudulent evasion of income tax". Her husband, Tim Whyte, is suspected of acting as a shadow director and is also being investigated in connection with the same offences.

Furthermore, two officials working in the VIP lane during the pandemic claim another politically connected PPE supplier – Bunzl was also dealt with via the VIP lane, also known as the High Priority Lane.

Bunzl had long been affiliated with Conservative peer Lord Feldman, who was also working as an advisor to health ministers during the pandemic.

Speaking to the inquiry this month Andy Wood, a deputy director and commercial specialist working for the Cabinet Office, said Bunzl was a "significant, credible offer" that was dealt with via the VIP lane after coming "into contact with the government via ministers and senior officials".

Wood's claim was supported by another senior civil servant, Max Cairnduff, who stated during his hearing on 6 March 2025 that Bunzl was a "really good lead" that potentially came into the VIP lane.

Gavin Hayman of the UKACC said: "I am not sure who is right but it is bad that we still don't know for sure five years on" the true extent of the VIP lane.

He urged the Inquiry to establish the true picture by "conducting a comprehensive review of the scale of and outcomes from the VIP Lane".

So far, the names of 51 recipients of the VIP lane have been published by the government, but this could be woefully short with potentially a further 22 PPE suppliers missing from the list.[4]

Company that supplied hundreds of millions of pounds of unusable Covid tests saw profits skyrocket to £178 million after lobbying Conservative peer for contract – published 28 April 2025

A company that was placed on the 'VIP' priority route for Covid contracts under the last Conservative government saw their profits soar to £178 million after successfully lobbying a senior Conservative peer to help them secure a contract for hundreds of millions of pounds worth of coronavirus tests that were later deemed mostly unusable.

Financial records reveal that Southampton-based company Primer Design Ltd, owned by French parent company Novacyt, had a bumper year during the first year of Covid. Its turnover in 2019 was £5.5 million, but following the award of two huge VIP contracts from the Department for Health and Social Care (DHSC) in 2020, this ballooned to £273 million of which £178 million was declared as profit. Two of the firms' directors received bonuses of £8.5 million and £3 million.

Accounts filed by Primer Design brag that sales "grew by over 4,800%" driven "principally" by its UK government contracts.

Primer Design was awarded its first £63 million contract by the DHSC in April 2020; this was followed by a £406 million deal in September 2020 – a two-year contract to supply PCR Covid tests.

According to analysis by *Private Eye*, Primer Design recorded a profit margin of 65.3% during the first Covid period, which led to them occupying the top spot in its league table of profitable pandemic contract winners.

Private Eye noted that Primer Design's profit margins were "double the world's most profitable company and creator of the most in demand 'intellectual property', Apple, and three times that achieved by Google".

The contracts ended in disaster after the DHSC deemed the testing kits supplied by Primer Design to be "unfit for public use" and lacking the "robustness" required. The majority of the kits were never used – resulting in the UK government attempting to seek a £145 million refund from Primer Design and its parent company, Novacyt, via the UK courts.

Both firms rejected the claims made by the DHSC and tried to countersue the government, eventually reaching an out-of-court settlement in June last year.

Questions still remained about how the firm was able to secure its place on the VIP lane. However, documents released to *Byline Times* now shed new light on this matter.

Lord Bethell held three meetings with executives from Novacyt on 4 April 2020 and 6 April 2020 to discuss the firm's Covid-19 testing capabilities – meetings that the Conservative peer failed to declare until June 2021, some 14 months later, as first reported by *Byline Times*.

However, emails disclosed to *Byline Times* via the Freedom of Information Act show that former Health Minister, Lord Bethell, was in regular correspondence with Novacyt and Primer Design in the days before the company landed its first VIP lane contract in April 2020.

Here's what the emails reveal:

✦ Following a telephone meeting between Lord Bethell and Novacyt, the firm emailed Lord Bethell attaching a memo containing a series of requests where "the Government can help Novacyt" as it begins "scaling up of the COVID-19 testing requirements". The four-page document seeks help on a broad range of issues including "financial support" from the DHSC as well as help with logistics. The firm also suggested the government could provide "an immediate injection of £5million".

✦ The informal email concluded with Novacyt officials suggesting to Bethell that "now it's time to light the BBQ and grab an hour of sunshine". The email received a response within half an hour and a follow up call was organised for the following day.

✦ Lord Bethell thanked Novacyt for the "very helpful note" before looping in another Conservative peer, Lord Andrew Fledman, to the email chain. Lord Feldman was operating as an advisor to health ministers during this time and controversially helped refer numerous companies onto the VIP lane.

✦ The firm also requested Lord Bethell's office issue a letter to Novacyt to acknowledge "the efforts" of Novacyt and Primer Design staff. Bethell obliged on the same day with a handwritten note embellished with the House of Lords letterhead, reading: "On behalf of the DHSC, I want to thank everyone at Novacyt for the remarkable contribution you are making in the fight against Coronavirus. It is recognised at the highest levels. And massively appreciated. Your ever, Lord Bethell."

✦ Novacyt officials lobbied Lord Bethell directly via email

again on 15 April 2020 and 20 April 2020 and in the subsequent months regarding products it could offer the DHSC, with Bethell noting in response that he had "played this into our recently upgraded system and will get back to you".

Novacyt's sustained lobbying efforts paid off, and on 26 April 2020 the company was awarded its first, £63 million contract from the DHSC, on the same day company executives emailed Lord Bethell and officials in the Cabinet Office thanking them for "your confidence and support". Bethell replied the following morning claiming "this is truly great news".

Primer Design Ltd and the DHSC were both contacted for comment.[5]

Civil servants felt pressured into giving 'special treatment' to Conservative-connected Covid PPE suppliers – published 21 March 2025

Civil servants felt pressured into giving "special treatment" to PPE suppliers with political connections to Conservative ministers, correspondence released by the Covid Inquiry has revealed.

The Inquiry this week heard from a civil servant tasked with procuring PPE from the suppliers that were referred to the unlawful VIP Lane during the pandemic.

The witness statement and accompanying evidence provided by Dawn Matthias-Jackson paints a damning picture of the political interference inherent at the time.

As the then-Conservative government scrambled to replenish stocks of masks, gloves and gowns during the early months of the pandemic in 2020, they set up a system which effectively fast-tracked bids from companies that had connections to the party. These contracts were inflated by at least £925 million, with VIP lane suppliers paid 80% more per unit than other suppliers.

In an email sent in May 2020, Mathias-Jackson suggests a member of the public should submit a Freedom of Information (FOI) request to ascertain how many VIP lane suppliers had "party connections", stating that in her opinion "it would be on the high side based on what I have seen going on".

This was in response to another civil servant describing the situation as, "Definitely a thing for mates... lots of back-scratching!"

There were also numerous eye-watering emails where civil servants voiced concerns over political pressure and the risk of escalation to ministers if they didn't respond to VIP suppliers promptly.

Emails published by the inquiry found:

+ In April 2020, civil servants were concerned by the "noise" from one unnamed VIP supplier who was threatening "escalation to Lord Feldman" because officials were taking too long completing the necessary due-diligence process – the pressure appeared to pay off and the offer was processed "ASAP". *Byline Times* has previously reported on Lord Feldman's involvement in lobbying officials on behalf of a PPE supplier, who was also a "good friend" of cabinet minister Michael Gove.
+ In an email sent on 31 March 2020, just one week into the first national lockdown, officials flagged the risk of VIP suppliers complaining to Boris Johnson, Matt Hancock and Gove if they didn't respond promptly enough to the supplier.

+ Civil servants felt "totally swamped" by the number of VIP cases that kept coming in and despite working up to 15 hours per day could not keep up with the "volume of emails".

+ According to officials, VIP suppliers "believed they are too important to complete a survey" that every other prospective PPE supplier outside of the VIP lane had to complete. Instead, they opted to utilise links to ministers or lobby Hancock or Gove and officials became nervous of the "noise" these suppliers could make if they were not contacted within 24 hours.

The evidence provided by Matthias-Jackson reveals she was worried by the "unfair" behaviour of a PPE supplier named Andrew Morris who claimed to have close ties to former Conservative Party minister Robert Jenrick.

In her statement to the Inquiry, Matthias-Jackson states: "I was concerned about Mr Morris because his persistence was extreme and he threatened to report me to Mr Jenrick when he met him later that evening in one phone call. I thought his behaviour was unfair."

Matthias-Jackson also claimed to have asked officials to "prioritise" certain VIP suppliers where she was receiving "pressure" and considered it possible that suppliers who had access to the high priority lane did receive "special treatment" because of the speed in which their offers were reviewed when compared to the thousands of other suppliers stuck in the public-facing procurement channels.[6]

Matt Hancock intervened to help Conservative donor's pizza firm land lucrative Covid PE contract – published 11 April 2025

Conservative former health secretary Matt Hancock personally helped top secure a Covid PPE contract for a former pizza company controlled by a Conservative donor, newly released documents reveal.

NKD International, owned by George Farha, repeatedly lobbied Hancock prior to securing a £135,000 PPE contract from the Department for Health and Social Care.

Farha had personally donated £11,450 to the Conservative Party and a further £12,500 to it via another company he controls.

The company had no record of previously supplying medical equipment and remarkably, just two days prior to the successful contract award, on 15 April 2020, it changed its name from 'NKD Pizza International Limited' to 'NKD International Limited' – dropping any reference to its previous record of selling fast food.

According to official records, NKD International was referred to the VIP lane by Dame Donna Kinnair, formerly of the Royal College of Nursing (RCN). Reports from 2021 reveal Kinnair was suspended from the RCN "amid concerns over her friendship with a multi-millionaire businessman" – George Farha.

Kinnair repeatedly lobbied Hancock via text message and email regarding Farha's NKD International's offer to supply medical gowns – with Hancock replying to one message stating: "Get him to email me again with the problems – I am working on this directly."

Farha's firm also tried to secure a second multi-million-pound PPE deal via the VIP lane, but was unsuccessful.

Documents provided to the Covid Inquiry reveal Hancock's close involvement:

+ On 11 April 2020, Kinnair had previously sent multiple WhatsApp messages to Hancock introducing Farha. One stated: "George Farha one of your party donators and my friend can get FDA approved gowns here by Wednesday."

+ According to Kinnair, on 13 April 2020, Hancock "replied by text message and asked me to get Mr Farha to contact him directly – four days later NKD International secured its VIP lane deal from the DHSC.

+ On 22 April 2020, according to the witness statement of health officials and less than one week after NKD secured its first PPE contract: "Mr Farha put forward an offer to supply 7.5 million sterile and non sterile gowns from Anhui Medpurest. The offer was to deliver 250,000 gowns per week over a period of 30 weeks on condition of a 50% advance payment per shipment." However, the offer ran into problems as NKD struggled to provide the correct certification for the PPE and officials raised concerns over the financial risks associated with the deal.

+ On 23 April 2020 Kinnair messaged Hancock and said: "I have to tell you after George has secured a regular supply with China at a fantastic price he is now being given the usual bureaucratic nonsense. With absurd scenarios being suggested. He has delivered and I am always unsure if those around are supporting your endeavours to get gowns and other PPE to the frontline."

+ According to Kinnair's Witness Statement to the Inquiry, Hancock replied saying: "Get him to email me again with the problems, I am working on this directly"

✦ Hancock repeatedly chased officials regarding the progress of the NKD International offer and also spoke directly with the firm.

Officials highlighted to the Inquiry the "completely atypical" nature of the NKD International contract process, due specifically to the "interest taken by the Secretary of State for Health, Matt Hancock MP".

NKD International was dissolved in June 2022 and could not be reached for comment.

It comes after *Byline Times* also revealed in a previous article 'Matt Hancock used his personal email account to help "VIP" supplier win £25 million Covid PPE contract'. Excalibur Healthcare, which supplied the UK government with tens of millions of pounds worth of unusable PPE, ultimately folded owing taxpayers £22 million.[7]

Conservative peer Lord Feldman helped 'good friend' of Michael Gove win VIP PPE deal – published 7 March 2025

The full extent of former Conservative Party chairman Lord Feldman's involvement in the PPE VIP lane scandal during the pandemic has been exposed by new documents released by the Covid Inquiry.

Records released to Good Law Project, following a lengthy Freedom of Information request battle in 2021, had already revealed that Feldman had referred three suppliers on the VIP lane – also known as the High Priority Lane. These firms (SG recruitment, Maxima Markets and Skinny Dip) then went on to secure lucrative PPE contracts from the former Conservative government.

However, the Covid Inquiry has now published documents

that suggest the Conservative Peer's involvement in the VIP lane scandal was much more extensive.

Feldman was 'secretly' hired by the Department of Health and Social Care in early 2020 to advise ministers on PPE procurement. It has now been revealed that he lobbied officials on multiple occasion on behalf of another VIP lane supplier, Meller Designs – owned by Conservative Party donor David Meller and long-time acquaintance of former cabinet minister Michael Gove.

Furthermore, evidence published by the Inquiry suggests Feldman referred a further 18 companies onto the VIP lane – albeit they didn't subsequently secure a deal.

Here's what the new evidence reveals:

+ On 3 April 2020, Lord Feldman and Lord Bethell emailed civil servants working in the VIP lane to chase progress on an offer of FFP3 face masks by Meller Designs. The company's owner, David Meller, has donated circa £60,000 to the Conservative Party. According to records, Feldman stated in his email that Mr Meller was "a good friend of Michael Gove".

+ In early May 2020, Feldman came to Meller's rescue again after civil servants had raised concerns over the suitability of IIR masks being proposed by Meller Designs. According to a witness statement published by the inquiry, the firm needed to obtain approval from the Medicines and Healthcare Products Regulatory Agency (MHRA), known as a 'derogation' to allow the masks to be used in the NHS. Feldman lobbied officials at the Cabinet Office to "expedite the process".

+ Feldman's private secretary also liaised directly with officials at the MHRA to ensure the "derogation request receive their

immediate attention". Two weeks later "a contract for the type IIR masks was subsequently awarded" to Meller Designs.
+ Meller Designs went on to secure six PPE contracts via the VIP lane worth circa £160 million in value.

The true extent of Lord Feldman's influence over civil servants in the VIP lane has started to emerge from the Covid Inquiry. A witness statement provided by a Cabinet Office civil servant provided explosive new evidence, namely:

+ Lord Feldman was involved in the referral of three companies to the HPL who later received contracts, and "referred at least 18 other companies to the HPL that did not receive contracts"
+ The inquiry documents list the new companies as follows: "Aquanima, Ben Gerbi Consulting, BHA Medical, Covaflu, FOSROC International, JDM Global Retail Solution, JHT Group, Lancea Partners, Mary Gorman, Next Pharma International, Nick Mason, Padma Textiles HK, Protector Plus LLC, Rostam Capital, Rowena Johnson, SGH Global, Suttersmill and The Hut Group."
+ The civil servant goes on to note: "As might be expected of a former party chair, some of his referrals had some connection to the Conservative Party but others did not." This included two firm linked "linked to Ben Elliott, then Chair of the Conservative Party" and another company FOSROC International "linked to Jim Hay, a party donor".
+ *Byline Times* revealed that Conservative party fixer Lord Feldman had lobbied Boris Johnson to push through a ventilator contract for Dyson. Private messages between Boris Johnson and his team reveal they were "on a mission" to secure the contract with leading Brexiteer James Dyson.[8]

Private correspondence reveals how David Cameron helped old Etonian school friend fast-track Covid testing firm – published 1 May 2025

Correspondence released to *Byline Times* reveals how former prime minister David Cameron helped an old Etonian school friend and former hedge funder get a fast track into the Department of Health and Social Care (DHSC) advisors at the start of the pandemic.

The friend was Hugh Warrender, who attended Eton with Cameron in the 1980s and who was then representing a South Korean Covid testing firm. After being contacted by Warrender, Cameron introduced him to Lord Feldman, another close friend of Cameron's, who was working as an advisor to health ministers at the time.

Knightsbridge based consultancy firm, Fin De Guerre Strategies, owned by Warrender, was ultimately unsuccessful in securing the contract for their clients from the DHSC. However, the company's "referral" from Cameron sheds new light on how businesses backed by senior Conservative Party figures were able to circumnavigate the usual procurement process.

Emails released to *Byline Times* via a Freedom of Information request reveal how within three days of lobbying the former PM, Fin De Guerre's offer to supply South Korean produced Covid tests was emailed directly to health minister Lord Bethell.

In the early hours of 3 April 2020, Cameron received an email from representatives of Fin De Guerre, the subject header of the email read: "Need your help — I have a supplier of COVID-19 tests but we can't contact anyone who replies to offer them."

The email included a plea to help provide contact details

for somebody in government with the "wherewithal to address" their offer to supply Covid tests "seriously".

Later the same morning, Cameron obliged and forwarded the offer on to Lord Feldman – a Conservative peer who was also working as an advisor to Matt Hancock and Lord Bethell during the early months of the pandemic.

Cameron told the supplier: "Hi there. Try Andrew Feldman – an old friend of mine and my former party chairman who runs a business but is currently working in the NHS, for Matt Hancock, sorting out various procurements". Cameron signed off the email "All good wishes. Dc."

The day after Cameron's introduction to the Conservative peer, the supplier emailed Lord Feldman directly on what appears to be his personal email address rather than his official DHSC account to request Feldman give its submission "more prompt attention".

Remarkably, within three hours Lord Feldman replied: "Thanks for this – you are doing all of the right things. We are getting a lot of offers of tests from South Korea at the moment as well as a huge volume of other offers. My job is to triage many of these offers across testing kits, ventilators, medicines and PPE for DHSC for Matthew Hancock and James Bethell."

Feldman, described as Cameron's oldest political friend, passed Fin De Guerre's Covid testing offer on to health minister and fellow Conservative peer Lord Bethell the next day on 5 April 2020.

Lord Bethell replied within 15 minutes of receiving the email from Lord Feldman, an email which was given the subject header "referral from David Cameron".

In his response Lod Bethell complained: "I just had a shocking procurement call. We need to think of ways around procurement."

Although Fin De Guerre's attempt to supply Covid tests to the DHSC appears to have not succeeded, the emails reveal how a supplier with a Conservative Party-backed "referral" was able to go from being ignored by civil servants to the front of the queue – all within the space of three days.

The DHSC, Cameron, Feldman and Warrender were all approached for comment. None responded by the time this article was published.[9]

What the experts suggest

Many NGOs, government committees and watchdogs have analysed the government's record on procurement and links to cronyism during the pandemic and published a host of sensible recommendations that could be enforced to ensure the consequences of past procurement and lobbying scandals are not repeated.

For the remainder of this chapter I will share the findings and recommendations from these respected organisations.

The Boardman reviews

Following a growing number of political scandals including the revelations over David Cameron's extensive lobbying campaign on behalf of Greensill Capital, the Cabinet Office recruited Nigel Boardman to investigate how the government handles the problems with conflicts of interests that arise when politicians operate between the private sector and their roles in Parliament.

The Boardman report was published on the 5 August 2021 and made a number of recommendations and suggestions. Those recommendations relevant to lobbying and transparency were as follows:[10]

Section I
Individuals' engagement, activities and terms of engagement with government

Recommendations

1. That government should establish an effective method for ensuring compliance with governance processes and the wider regulatory framework.
2. That government should introduce pre-appointment rules which prevent for a period of time civil servants dealing with or promoting their former employer after joining the civil service.
3. That government should further improve the management and monitoring of conflicts of interest in the Civil Service.
4. That government should strengthen whistleblowing processes in the Civil Service.
5. That direct ministerial appointments, whether or not remunerated, need a clearer and more transparent process, set out in a new Code of Practice which makes clear the expectations on both departments and appointees and reaffirms that express ministerial approval is required.
6. That government strengthens the oversight of the honours process within departments.

Suggestions

That government should establish a regular cycle of compliance reviews.
That the Code of Conduct for Board Members of Public Bodies and the Corporate Governance Code for central government departments should be given a statutory basis.
That government should consider introducing rules for securities dealings by civil servants.

Section 3
The relationship between current and former ministers and officials and external organisations
Recommendations
9. That government undertakes a follow up review to the Baxendale Report reviewing the experience of external hires into the Civil Service to ensure that impediments to effective recruitment and retention are eliminated, and that this exercise be repeated at regular intervals.
10. That the application process for secondary employment for civil servants should be more transparent and clearly regulated.
11. That government makes post-employment restrictions on civil servants and ministers legally binding.
12. That government develops with ACoBA a Memorandum of Understanding that sets out more clearly how they can work more effectively together.

Section 4

Engagement with government by those acting for and on behalf of external organisations

Recommendations

13. That government strengthens its transparency reporting by: – requiring more frequent returns; – defining more clearly what should be included in the return, including a sufficient explanation to enable a reader reasonably to be able to understand the purpose of the meeting and who was present at it; – designating a senior responsible departmental official who is properly trained to supervise the transparency returns; – reporting in their annual report on the timeliness of the publication of its transparency returns; and – requiring accounting officers to explain to their responsible Select Committees any failure to publish transparency returns in a timely manner.

14. That government extends the definition of 'meeting' to include all forms of non-public interactive dialogue which, were it face to face, would constitute a meeting requiring inclusion in the transparency return.

15. That government publishes an appropriate set of principles to define when an interactive communication should be deemed official business and therefore disclosed.

16. That the requirement to register as a consultant lobbyist should be extended: – to lobbyists employed by more than one organisation; – to any former senior civil servant or minister who engages in lobbying; – by removing or severely curtailing the exemption for 'incidental lobbying'; and – by removing the exemption for those not registered for VAT.

17. That the rules regarding the transparency of lobbyists be strengthened by:
 – requiring lobbyists to disclose the ultimate person paying for, or benefiting from, their lobbying activity;
– lobbyists including in their quarterly information returns the number of incidents of lobbying, the subject matter in sufficient detail for a third party to understand the nature of the lobbying, and which named individuals were lobbied;
– requiring registered lobbyists to meet a statutory code of conduct, setting minimum standards;
– government keeping under review whether the Registrar of Lobbyists should be able to impose more meaningful penalties for non-compliance, particularly in the event a statutory code of conduct (which seeks to police behaviour) is introduced; and making knowingly deceiving in the process of lobbying a criminal offence.

18. That government impose a contractual prohibition on contractors referring to government contracts in marketing material without government consent.

19. That government requires tenderers to disclose any former minister or senior civil servant employed or retained by them and explain the steps they have taken to ensure that they have not thereby obtained an unfair advantage in a procurement exercise.

The recommendations made within the Boardman review were welcomed by the Institute for Government, which said: "Boardman's suggestions are wide-ranging and ambitious. If implemented they will represent a sea-change in how government manages real and perceived conflicts of interest". The organisation also sounded the alarm regarding the government's desire to enforce the recommendations made by Boardman. Unfortunately at the time of writing the government seems to have broadly ignored the contents of the report.[11]

Boardman was also recruited to conduct a "short and targeted review" of government procurement during the pandemic – again following the growing number of political scandals engulfing the government and its procurement of medical equipment.

Boardman made 28 key recommendations that urged the government to "improve contingency planning for future pandemics". Boardman suggested the NHS procurement teams should in future, maintain "supply chain maps" that allow for PPE to be purchased directly from manufacturers rather than through a controversial intermediary ("distributor"). Boardman also argued that "spend controls should still apply in times of crisis" and if the government appoints an external advisor to lead on key programmes then a senior civil servant should also be identified to work in "parallel" with them.[12]

Spotlight on Corruption

In December 2020, the NGO Spotlight on Corruption, whose work is referenced in this book, made a number of recommendations that would improve the way the government could manage conflict of interests risk when making big procurement decisions. The anti-corruption organisation suggested:[13]

Recommendation 1	"Urgently establish a centralised function to record and manage conflicts of interests in government, in line with UN and GRECO recommendations"
Recommendation 2	"Conduct a full review of outstanding conflicts of interest in Covid contracts, and ensure these are made public and a road map for how they are being managed laid out"
Recommendation 3	"Ensure that going forward, all contracts awarded meet standards laid out in Regulation 24 of the Public Contracts Regulations, with a full paper trail of decisions made, and full transparency of how conflicts of interest have been handled"
Recommendation 4	"Review with immediate effect the remit of the Independent Advisor on ministers Interests in line with UN and GRECO recommendations, to give the Advisor independent statutory status including power to investigate conflicts of interest by ministers and to take action if required."

Transparency International

In April 2021, Transparency International (TI), a leading non-governmental anti-corruption organisation, published its report titled 'Track and Trace: Identifying corruption risks in UK public procurement from the Covid-19 pandemic'.

TI's decision to investigate the contentious procurement decision followed the organisation observing a worrying pattern of behaviour "whereby critical safeguards for protecting the public purse have been thrown aside without adequate justification". Following the investigation TI made ten recommendations that it considered would improve the current situation and avoid future corruption risks.[14]

Competitive ten- dering and crisis contracting	Recommendation 1 The public sector should now be back to undertaking competitive procurement as a default.
	Recommendation 2 Truncated procurement processes should be limited only to declared emergencies under a new power that has been proposed by the UK government. Orders made under this power should be: • the principal legal basis for truncated procurement during a crisis period • limited to procurement relating to the immediate requirements of the crisis response • still require full transparency of any contract awards during the crisis period within the standard publica- tion deadlines Any order used should be subject to parliamentary oversight. This could involve an order being subject to: • the made affirmative procedure in at most two instances within a year, with parliamentary approval of the order within 28 days of the order being laid • a sunset clause of up to 90 days • any subsequent renewal requiring the minister to make a statement before the House explaining why it is necessary, and an affirmative procedure • a statutory review ending no more than 12 months after the end of the last crisis period declared under these power
Transparency and accounta- bility over the VIP lane	Recommendation 3 The award of the 73 contracts we identify in this report should be subject to detailed audits by the rel- evant authorities. The UK government should provide clarity over the current status of the VIP lane and end it if it has not done so already. To provide greater assurance and accountability on the matter, the UK government should also provide transparency of the: • names of the companies referred to the VIP lane • source of the referral • decision for the referral • status of the referral • any conflicts of interest identified for these referrals

Managing bribery and corruption risks in crisis procurement	**Recommendation 4** The UK government should work to ensure there is a robust stockpile and supply chain of PPE to deal with future pandemic crises, and provide a progress update to Parliament on their implementation by July 2021.
	Recommendation 5 Public bodies should clearly incorporate bribery and corruption risk assessments and mitigation strategies into their procurement practices for crisis responses
Transparency and access to information	**Recommendation 6** The Minister for the Cabinet Office should make a statement to Parliament setting out: • where the UK government has not complied with its legal transparency obligations under the Public Contracts Regulations 2015 and FOIA, • how these are being rectified, and • how departments will prevent the same issues recurring in the future
Improve public procurement practice going forward	**Recommendation 7** The UK government should include its proposals to require company identifiers in procurement and spend data as part of its forthcoming reforms of public procurement
	Recommendation 8 The UK government should include its measures to improve the quality and consistency of data in its forthcoming reforms of public procurement, including single identities for buyers and suppliers, and controls on data entry by contracting authorities
Deterrents against potential misconduct	**Recommendation 9** Responsibility for overseeing and enforcing the ministerial code should be moved to an office independent of government with sufficient powers and resources to undertake their role effectively. The position should be appointed, resourced by, and accountable to Parliament.
	Recommendation 10 The UK government should bring forward legislation for a new statutory offence of corruption in public office at the earliest possible opportunity.

The Public Accounts Committee

The Public Accounts Committee's 42nd report, titled 'Covid-19: Government procurement and supply of Personal Protective Equipment' and published on 10 February 2021, highlighted a number of concerns about the government's management and procurement of PPE goods during the pandemic. Chaired by Labour MP Meg Hillier and supported by 15 other MPs from across the political spectrum, the committee made seven suggestions to the government:[15]

1	Transparency: "Government should ensure all the Boardman review recommendations are applied across government departments and procuring bodies. The Cabinet Office should write to us by July 2021 outlining its progress in implementing the recommendations of the Boardman review and a timetable for implementing any outstanding recommendations".
2	Stockpile of PPE: "The Department must improve its approach to managing and distributing stocks of PPE to ensure the correct equipment gets to those who need it, when they need it. The Department should write to us by July 2021 to confirm that: • Stockpiles hold everything required as specified in the Department's plans. • Stock is checked regularly and there is a process for monitoring and replacing stock before it is out-of-date. • Stock is held in locations from which it can be distributed quickly when required • There are contingency plans to secure new items of clinical equipment which may be needed at short notice".
3	High Priority Lane: "The Cabinet Office and the Department should by July 2021 publish the lessons it has learnt from the procurement of PPE during the pandemic for future emergencies and disseminate these lessons to the wider government commercial function. This should include guidance for determining what is considered a credible offer and how this is communicated to potential suppliers".
4	Social Care: "The Department should write to the Committee by the end of April 2021 to explain how it will revise its emergency response plans so that they include who will be supported, how and when. This must give appropriate weight to all sectors of health and social care, as well as occupations outside these sectors which are also at risk".

5	BAME staff: "The Department needs to better understand the experience of frontline staff during the first wave of the pandemic, and ensure lessons are learned so it can better respond in a future emergency. It should particularly focus on the different reported experiences of staff from different ethnic backgrounds and consider how this should be monitored and tackled in future – not just in a pandemic. It should write to us by July 2021 setting out the results of this work and how these lessons are being applied. This work should cover: • How many health and social care providers ran out of each type of PPE during the pandemic. • Why many health and social care staff reported shortages of PPE, whereas the organisations they worked for did not appear to report shortages. • The extent to which (and reasons why) BAME staff were less likely to report having access to PPE and being tested for PPE, and more likely to report feeling pressured to work without adequate PPE. • Whether there are any links between PPE shortages and staff infections and deaths (when the relevant investigations have completed), including the deaths of health and care workers who do not work in NHS trusts. • Provider organisations' and frontline staff views on PPE guidance".
6	Over-ordering of PPE: "The Department, working with other government departments where necessary, should set out a plan by July 2021 that shows how it will: • Use the PPE it has ordered, covering how much will be given health and social care providers, stockpiled, cancelled, or sold in the UK or overseas. • Incentivise the NHS Supply Chain, trusts and other providers, to buy PPE which is made in the UK. • Ensure there is sufficient resilience in the supply chain where UK manufacturers cannot provide the necessary PPE".
7	PPE quality checks: "The Department should write to the Committee by July 2021 setting out how much of the PPE it ordered it has received and checked, and the volumes and costs of the PPE that (a) cannot be used at all; (b) cannot be used for its intended purpose; and (c) its methodology for determining the volumes and costs of PPE which it considers to be in each of these categories"

The National Audit Office

Throughout the pandemic the NAO has issued a number of scathing reports following its examination of PPE contracts, ventilator procurement and the Covid testing programme. With regard to PPE procurement, in December 2020, the NAO suggested six lessons to be learned that could improve future government decision-making:[16]

A	The Department and its partners had to oversee and take many unplanned and unprecedented actions to obtain PPE during the emergency. Inevitably, some actions were more successful than others. A comprehensive lessons-learned exercise involving all the main stakeholders, including local government and representatives of the workforce and suppliers, would inform the planning for future emergencies. This should include: consideration of whether any issues with PPE provision or use might have contributed to Covid-19 infections or deaths; how to determine the priorities when there are shortages of essential equipment such as PPE; and, how events are recorded during an emergency response to help learn lessons for the future.
B	Business-as-usual activities within government need to strike the appropriate balance between operational and financial efficiency versus the longer-term need for resilience and capability for dealing with shocks. For PPE, this includes consideration of the cost implications of, and incentives needed for, developing and maintaining a domestic manufacturing base and increasing diversity in international supply.
C	Emergency plans for dealing with a pandemic must provide for appropriate stockpiles of high-quality PPE together with comprehensive and resilient arrangements for the rapid procurement and distribution of PPE, based on reliable information. Plans need to include distribution of PPE to social care and all parts of the health system. Organisations responsible for maintaining and testing their plans must actively monitor for new threats that might overwhelm their plans.
D	Effective governance, lines of accountability, and resourcing responsibilities are important for an effective rapid response in an emergency situation. Developing these arrangements, and ensuring that they remain up to date, should be part of the emergency plan for activation when required.

E	Clear, timely, two-way information and communication are vital for both providing services at the front-line and for managing the response at the national level. This includes information on national and local PPE stocks and requirements, and feedback loops. Deficiencies in information on, and communication about, PPE can lead to a breakdown of trust, failure to take effective action, and poor value for money.
F	Despite efforts to integrate them over the years, health and social care have continued to be separate systems. During this crisis the social care sector was hit hard by shortages of PPE, and government needs to understand why national bodies provided more support to hospitals than to social care and how to prevent that happening again.

Chapter 8

Afterword

By March 2022, the Office for Budget Responsibility (OBR), the watchdog established to monitor government fiscal policies, had estimated that the UK had spent £311 billion on "pandemic-related support measures" – the equivalent of handing £4,631 to every person in the UK. This was a figure that could rise to as much as £373 billion according to the NAO.[1]

His Majesty's Treasury has estimated that £96.7 billion was spent by the DHSC, which led on the flagship vaccination, PPE and Test and Trace programmes, wasting multiple billions of pounds procuring goods from dubious sources – often purchasing products that were not fit for purpose and excessively inflated in price.

As the government continues to incinerate billions of items of unusable PPE, millions of Brits are now grappling with the financial pressures of the current "cost of living" crisis. Many are struggling to pay their mortgages, rent, bills and groceries – a striking juxtaposition when compared to the individuals who grossly profited from the government's unlawful VIP lane. These individuals are now splashing the cash on private jets, super yachts, stately homes and luxurious overseas villas – a position many of the "VIP lane" recipients found themselves in not by merit, but because of the political connections they had within the governing Conservative Party.

A reported 227,000 people died in the UK as a result of Covid-19. This is a fact that shouldn't be forgotten when we also talk about the cronyism and corruption that overshadowed the Conservative government since Covid hit. Lessons must be learned. Never again should NHS staff have to wear bin bags to treat pandemic patients, putting their lives at risk simply because the UK hasn't procured the correct medical gowns for them to wear, ignoring reputable suppliers and instead throwing billions of pounds at unqualified peers and party donors, who ultimately fail to deliver, but are still allowed to retain the vast profits bestowed upon them.

One hard truth remains: no other country *in the world* established a special process to procure medical goods during the pandemic – just one more example of how the UK was a Covid outlier in all the wrong ways. Let's be as clear and straightforward as possible about what happened: the Conservative government set up a mechanism to prioritise bids for life-saving goods based not on value for your money, quality, track record or speed of delivery. No, the Conservative government set up a mechanism to prioritise bids based on a supplier's political connections. It's that simple. And it's that shameful. It will forever be a decision that cost the country dearly not just in financial terms but in human lives.

Acknowledgements

Writing this book was half a decade in the making, a task that would have been impossible without the unwavering support and encouragement from my wife, Harri. While I was investigating dodgy PPE contracts, she was raising our two amazing children – Frankie and Finn, both of whom have provided moments of joy whilst drafting the book (interrupting countless Zoom calls in the process).

Special thanks to my agent Euan Thorneycroft at A M Heath for his invaluable assistance throughout. Writing a book of this nature can create many obstacles and I'm grateful for Euan's support as we navigate our way through them.

I am thankful to my publishers – *Byline Books*, in particular Peter Jukes, Stephen Colegrave and Ella Baddeley for their unwavering support and Kyle Taylor for his talented editing, ideas and patience. Also a big thanks to James Vaughan-Jones at Reviewed and Cleared and Mark Ecob at Mecob Designs.

I was incredibly lucky to land my dream job at Good Law Project during the pandemic and I owe a huge thanks to my former boss Jolyon Maugham KC who encouraged and supported me whilst I investigated this subject for three years and whose passion for fighting for transparency has been inspiring. I also appreciate the teamwork and support of my former colleagues at GLP, in particular Tim Picton, Rachel Smethers and Gemma Abbott.

I have been lucky enough to collaborate with some of the best investigative journalists and researchers in the country while investigating the VIP lane, many of whom have provided me with invaluable experience and inspired me to keep digging – in particular Peter Geoghegan, David Conn, Nic Sommerlad and Steve Goodrich.

Working freelance can be daunting at times. I am very grateful for the support, kindness and amplification of my work by Carol Vorderman and James O'Brien as well as the team at *Byline Times*.

A big thank you to Brian Wood, Rachel Watson, Davina Bristow, Jenna Weiler and Will Hecker at Truevision and Tom Giles at ITV for believing in the project and turning the story into a TV documentary. It's a dream come true to write a book and work on a documentary.

It would have been almost impossible to write this book without the bravery and knowledge shared by the many sources that provided me with valuable insight. I cannot name them here – but they know who they are.

I am deeply grateful to my family, in particular my mum, dad, my twin brother Kevin, my two sisters Tracey and Jayne, Gill, Ivan, Lauren, Rob, Maria, Sandy and Phil, and to my friends Sam, Pete and Daryl, who have always supported me while i researched, investigated and wrote this book (and who have had to endure me ranting about PPE and Test and Trace for five years).

Finally, in memory of my nan Joan, who sadly succumbed to Covid in late 2020, a truly inspiring grandmother and person, who certainly inspired me to continue my work.

Notes

Preface

1. Trust and confidence in Britain's system of government at record low. (2024, June 12). National Centre for Social Research. https://natcen. ac.uk/news/trust-and-confidence-britains-system-government-record-low

2. Brien P, Keep M, (2023, September 12). *Public spending during the Covid-19 pandemic.* House of Commons Library. https:// researchbriefings.files.parliament.uk/documents/CBP-9309/CBP-9309. pdf

3. Verity, A. (2024, September 9). *Corruption review finds 'red flags' in more than 130 Covid contracts.* BBC, https://www.bbc.co.uk/news/articles/ cevj3y7n33vo

4. Scott, (2024, February 2). *Michael Gove opened the door to biggest VIP lane firm.* Good Law Project. https://goodlawproject.org/michael-gove-opened-the-door-to-biggest-vip-lane-firm/

Introduction

1. Giuffrida, A., & Tondo, L. (2020, February 24). Italians Struggle With 'surreal' Lockdown As Coronavirus Cases Rise. *The Guardian.* https:// www.theguardian.com/world/2020/feb/24/italians-struggle-with-surreal-lockdown-as-coronavirus-cases-rise

2. 'I Shook Hands With Everybody,' Says Boris Johnson Weeks Before Coronavirus Diagnosis – video. (2020, March 27). *The Guardian.* https:// www.theguardian.com/world/video/2020/mar/27/i-shook-hands-with-everybody-says-boris-johnson-weeks-before-coronavirus-diagnosis-video

3. Coronavirus: The World In Lockdown In Maps And Charts. (2020, April

6). BBC News. https://www.bbc.co.uk/news/world-52103747https:// www.bbc.co.uk/news/world-52103747

4. Cummings, D. (2023, October 12). INQ000273872 – Witness Statement Of Dominic Cummings Dated 12/10/2023. UK Covid-19 Inquiry Archives. UK Covid-19 Inquiry. https://covid19.public-inquiry.uk/ documents/inq000273872-witness-statement-of-dominic-cummings-dated-12-10-2023/

5. Scott, R., & Geoghegan, P. (2020, September 15). Revealed: Boris Johnson Under Fire Over 'personal' Meeting With Russian Oligarch During COVID-19 Pandemic. OpenDemocracy. https://www.opendemocracy.net/en/dark-money-investigations/ revealed-boris-johnson-under-fire-over-personal-meeting-with-russian-oligarch-during-covid-19-pandemic/

6. Prime Minister's Statement On Coronavirus (COVID-19): 23 March 2020. (2020, March 23). GOV.UK. https://www.gov.uk/government/ speeches/pm-address-to-the-nation-on-coronavirus-23-march-2020

7. Coronavirus disease 2019 (COVID-19) Situation Report – 63. (2020, March 23). World Health Organisation. https://www.who.int/docs/ default-source/coronaviruse/situation-reports/20200323-sitrep-63-covid-19.pdf

8. Scott, R., & Howard, E. (2020, July 23). Even After A Global Ban, Pangolins Are Still Legally Traded. Unearthed. https://unearthed. greenpeace.org/2020/07/23/pangolin-ban-legal-trade-cites-china-us/

9. Geoghegan, P., & Scott, R. (2020, October 9). Government Accused Of 'cronyism' After Tory Councillor Wins £156m COVID Contract. OpenDemocracy. https://www.opendemocracy.net/en/ dark-money-investigations/government-accused-of-cronyism-after-tory-councillor-wins-156m-covid-contract/

10. Pogrund, G. (2020, November 22). Tory Steve Dechan's £276m In PPE Contracts Lands Him A Place In The Country. The Times. https://www. thetimes.co.uk/article/tory-steve-dechans-276m-in-ppe-contracts-lands-him-a-place-in-the-country-zgbmmtn8q

11. Bright, S. (2020, September 18). Firm Owned By Conservative Donor Nets Additional £81.8 Million Government PPE Deals. Byline Times. https://bylinetimes.com/2020/09/18/firm-meller-designs-conservative-donor-nets-millions-government-ppe-deals/

12. The Electoral Commission. (2023, May 13). http://bit.ly/3JrTxgE

13. Geoghegan, P., & Scott, R. (2021, January 20). Tory Donor Lord Ashcroft's Outsourcing Firm Lands £350m Vaccination Contract. OpenDemocracy. https://www.opendemocracy.net/en/ dark-money-investigations/revealed-tory-donor-lord-ashcrofts-

outsourcing-firm-given-350m-vaccination-contract/

14. Geoghegan, P., & Scott, R. (2021, January 20). Tory Donor Lord Ashcroft's Outsourcing Firm Lands £350m Vaccination Contract. OpenDemocracy. https://www.opendemocracy.net/en/dark-money-investigations/revealed-tory-donor-lord-ashcrofts-outsourcing-firm-given-350m-vaccination-contract/

15. Exposed: Special Procurement Channels For 'VIPs' And Cabinet Contacts – Good Law Project. (2020, October 29). Good Law Project. https://goodlawproject.org/special-procurement-channels/

Chapter I: The VIP lane

1. Walker, P. (2021, November 11). Boris Johnson Says The UK Is Not 'remotely A Corrupt Country'. Is It? *The Guardian*. https://www.theguardian.com/politics/2021/nov/11/boris-johnson-says-the-uk-is-not-remotely-a-corrupt-country-is-it

2. The ABCs Of The CPI: How The Corruption Perceptions Index Is…. (2021, December 20). Transparency.Org. https://www.transparency.org/en/news/how-cpi-scores-are-calculated

3. 2023 Corruption Perceptions Index: Explore The Results. (2024, January 30). Transparency.Org. https://www.transparency.org/en/cpi/2023

4. Concerns Of Corruption At All-time High As UK Falls To Its Lowest Ever Score On Global Corruption Perceptions Index. (2024, January 30). Transparency International UK. https://www.transparency.org.uk/concerns-corruption-all-time-high-uk-falls-its-lowest-ever-score-global-corruption-perceptions-index

5. Government Must Get A Grip On Conflicts Of Interest In Public Procurement Or Risk Losing The UKs Reputation As A Fair Place To Do Business – Spotlight On Corruption. (2020, November 23). Spotlight on Corruption. https://www.spotlightcorruption.org/government-must-get-a-grip-on-conflicts-of-interest-in-public-procurement-or-risk-losing-the-uks-reputation-as-a-fair-place-to-do-business/

6. The supply of personal protective equipment (PPE) during the COVID-19 pandemic. (2020, November 25). National Audit Office. https://www.nao.org.uk/wp-content/uploads/2020/11/The-supply-of-personal-protective-equipment-PPE-during-the-COVID-19-pandemic.pdf

7. Mahmood, B. (2024, February 9). EXCLUSIVE: Nearly Half Of Voters Think Current Tory Government Is More Corrupt Than Previous Governments, Poll Finds. Left Foot Forward: Leading The UK's Progressive Debate. https://leftfootforward.org/2024/02/exclusive-nearly-half-of-voters-think-current-tory-government-is-more-

corrupt-than-previous-governments-poll-finds/

8. The supply of personal protective equipment (PPE) during the COVID-19 pandemic. (2020, November 25). National Audit Office. https://www.nao.org.uk/wp-content/uploads/2020/11/The-supply-of-personal-protective-equipment-PPE-during-the-COVID-19-pandemic.pdf

9. NQ000093009_0005-0007 – Extract Of Matt Hancock's WhatsApp Messages From Covid-19 Senior Group, Dated 25/01/2020. UK Covid-19 Inquiry Archives. (2024, February 16). UK Covid-19 Inquiry. https://covid19.public-inquiry.uk/documents/inq000093009_0005-0007-extract-of-matt-hancocks-whatsapp-messages-from-covid-19-senior-group-dated-25-01-2020/

10. Press, C. (2020, April 5). Coronavirus: The NHS Workers Wearing Bin Bags As Protection. BBC News. https://www.bbc.co.uk/news/health-52145140

11. Nearly Half Of England's Doctors Forced To Find Their Own PPE, Data Shows. (2020, May 3). *The Guardian*. https://www.theguardian.com/uk-news/2020/may/03/nearly-half-of-british-doctors-forced-to-find-their-own-ppe-new-data-shows

12. Campbell, D. (2020, April 27). UK Doctors Finding It Harder To Get PPE Kit To Treat Covid-19 Patients, Research Reveals. *The Guardian*. https://www.theguardian.com/society/2020/apr/27/uk-doctors-finding-it-harder-to-get-ppe-kit-to-treat-covid-19-patients-research-reveals

13. INQ000057530 – Government Internal Audit Agency. Draft Report Titled Department Of Health And Social Care, Analysis Of PPE Issue, Dated 21/09/2020 UK Covid-19 Inquiry Archives. (2020, September 21). UK Covid-19 Inquiry. https://covid19.public-inquiry.uk/documents/inq000057530-draft-report-titled-department-of-health-and-social-care-analysis-of-ppe-issue-dated-21-09-2020/

14. Davies, H. (2020, May 14). Drivers Tell Of Chaos At UK's Privately Run PPE Stockpile. *The Guardian*. https://www.theguardian.com/world/2020/may/14/coronavirus-uk-privately-run-ppe-stockpile-chaos-movianto

15. ITV News. (2020). Revealed: Insiders voice their concerns about management of PPE stockpile. ITV News https://www.youtube.com/watch?v=8YUa_3AxNQw

16. Campbell, Dennis. (2020, April 23). Emails Reveal Doctor's Plea For PPE Before Covid-19 Death. *The Guardian*. https://www.theguardian.com/society/2020/apr/23/emails-reveal-doctors-plea-for-ppe-before-covid-19-death-dr-peter-tun

17. Croxford, R. (2020, April 2). Coronavirus: NHS Worker 'let Down' Before Death. BBC News. https://www.bbc.co.uk/news/uk-england-london-52131921

Notes

18. Coronavirus (COVID-19) Related Deaths By Occupation, England And Wales – Office For National Statistics. (2021, January 25). Office for National Statistics. https://www.ons.gov.uk/peoplepopulationandcommunity/healthandsocialcare/causesofdeath/datasets/coronaviruscovid19relateddeathsbyoccupationenglandandwales

19. The supply of personal protective equipment (PPE) during the COVID-19 pandemic. (2020a, November 25). National Audit Office. https://www.nao.org.uk/wp-content/uploads/2020/11/The-supply-of-personal-protective-equipment-PPE-during-the-COVID-19-pandemic.pdf

20. COVID-19: Government procurement and supply of Personal Protective Equipment. Forty-Second Report of Session 2019–21. (2021, February 4). House of Commons Public Accounts Committee. https://committees.parliament.uk/publications/4607/documents/46709/default/

21. Investigation into the management of PPE contracts. (2022, March 30). National Audit Office. https://www.nao.org.uk/wp-content/uploads/2022/03/Investigation-into-the-management-of-PPE-contracts.pdf

22. Exposed: Special Procurement Channels For 'VIPs' And Cabinet Contacts – Good Law Project. (2020, October 29). Good Law Project. https://goodlawproject.org/special-procurement-channels/

23. Investigation into the management of PPE contracts. (2022, March 30). National Audit Office. https://www.nao.org.uk/wp-content/uploads/2022/03/Investigation-into-the-management-of-PPE-contracts.pdf

24. PPE Procurement VIP Lane – A Freedom Of Information Request To Cabinet Office. (2021, October 14). WhatDoTheyKnow. https://www.whatdotheyknow.com/request/ppe_procurement_vip_lane

25. Scott, R. (2021, June 30). NEW: Documents Reveal VIP Lane For Testing Contracts – Good Law Project. Good Law Project. https://goodlawproject.org/vip-lane-for-testing-contracts/

26. Pegg, D., Lawrence, F., & Conn, D. (2020, November 18). PPE Suppliers With Political Ties Given 'high-priority' Status, Report Reveals. *The Guardian*. https://www.theguardian.com/politics/2020/nov/18/ppe-suppliers-with-political-ties-given-high-priority-status-report-reveals

27. (2021, May 17). 2021.05.14 –[redacted] – PPE Hearing C Skeleton.pdf. Good Law Project. https://drive.google.com/file/d/1uaBqzBp9mntEg5ofM40m13NGS47MXDAg/view

28. Explosive Emails Show How The Government's VIP Lane Caused Chaos In PPE Procurement – Good Law Project. (2021, April 22). Good Law Project. https://goodlawproject.org/ppe-urgent-hearing/

29. Scott, R,. (2021, May 30). Twitter.com. https://twitter.com/russellscott1/status/1398951453792915456?lang=cs

30. Good Law Project,. (2021, April 29). Twitter.com,. https://x.com/GoodLawProject/status/1387736470098690051?s=20

31. (2021, May 17). 2021.05.14 –[redacted] – PPE Hearing C Skeleton.pdf. Good Law Project. https://drive.google.com/file/d/1uaBqzBp9mntEg5of M40m13NGS47MXDAg/view

32. The Guide to Freedom of Information. (2017, August 14). Information Commissioner's Office. https://ico.org.uk/media/for-organisations/guide-to-freedom-of-information-4-9.pdf

33. Geoghegan, P., Corderoy, J., & Amin, L. (2020, November 23). UK Government Running 'Orwellian' Unit To Block Release Of 'sensitive' Information. OpenDemocracy. https://www.opendemocracy.net/en/freedom-of-information/uk-government-running-orwellian-unit-to-block-release-of-sensitive-information/

34. Breaking: Government Ordered To Reveal The Names Of Companies In The PPE VIP Lane – Good Law Project. (2021, October 18). Good Law Project. https://goodlawproject.org/they-have-to-reveal-the-names/

35. (2021, October 18). ICO Decision Letter. Reference IC-94513-N5H8. Good Law Project. https://drive.google.com/file/d/1BAvBbnviHY3UOK LAxcP1JbBXY4KNIqKD/view

36. Scott, R. (2021b, November 16). LEAKED: The Conservative Politicians Who Referred Companies To The PPE 'VIP Lane' – Good Law Project. Good Law Project. https://goodlawproject.org/conservative-politicians-vip-lane/

37. Scott, R. (2021c, November 18). Revealed: Then There Were 50! Government Comes Clean About Three New "VIPs" – Good Law Project. Good Law Project. https://goodlawproject.org/revealed-then-there-were-50/

38. BREAKING: High Court Finds Government PPE 'VIP' Lane For Politically Connected Suppliers 'unlawful' – Good Law Project. (2022, January 12). Good Law Project. https://goodlawproject.org/update/high-court-vip-lane-ppe-unlawful/

39. PPE MEDPRO LIMITED Filing History – Find And Update Company Information – GOV.UK. (2024, May 15). Companies House. https://find-and-update.company-information.service.gov.uk/company/12597000/filing-history

40. Home – PPE Medpro. (2024, May 15). PPE Medpro. https://ppemedpro.com/

41. 41.Products – PPE Medpro. (2024, May 15). PPE Medpro. https://ppemedpro.com/products/

42. Supply Of Personal Protective Equipment For Healthcare Workers For The Care Of Patients With Suspected Or Confirmed Novel Coronavirus (COVID-19) – Contracts Finder. (2020, October 20). Contracts Finder, GOV.UK. https://www.contractsfinder.service.gov.uk/notice/782b70db-4a13-4f67-87a6-8f1a5030cae5?origin=SearchResults&p=1

43. Supply Of Personal Protective Equipment For Healthcare Workers For The Care Of Patients With Suspected Or Confirmed Novel Coronavirus (COVID-19) – Contracts Finder. (2020a, September 7). Contracts Finder, GOV.UK. https://www.contractsfinder.service.gov.uk/notice/79397607-466e-4891-b091-3307fd5819d9?origin=SearchResults&p=1

44. Sommerlad, N. (2020, October 7). Firm Run By Ex-associate Of Tory Peer Michelle Mone Wins £112million NHS Deal. *The Mirror*. https://www.mirror.co.uk/news/politics/firm-run-ex-associate-tory-22810575

45. Conn, D., Scott, R., & Pegg, D. (2020, December 21). Firm With Mystery Investors Wins £200m Of PPE Contracts Via 'high-priority Lane.' *The Guardian*. https://www.theguardian.com/world/2020/dec/21/firm-with-mystery-investors-wins-200m-of-ppe-contracts-via-high-priority-lane

46. Scott, R. (2021b, November 16). LEAKED: The Conservative Politicians Who Referred Companies To The PPE 'VIP Lane' – Good Law Project. Good Law Project. https://goodlawproject.org/conservative-politicians-vip-lane/

47. Davies, C., & Conn, D. (2023, December 17). How The Michelle Mone Scandal Unfolded: £200m Of PPE Contracts, Denials And A Government Lawsuit. *The Guardian*. https://www.theguardian.com/uk-news/2023/dec/17/how-the-michelle-mone-scandal-unfolded-200m-of-ppe-contracts-denials-and-a-government-lawsuit

48. Conn, D., Lewis, P., & Davies, H. (2022, January 6). Tory Peer Michelle Mone Secretly Involved In PPE Firm She Referred To Government. *The Guardian*. https://www.theguardian.com/world/2022/jan/06/tory-peer-michelle-mone-involved-ppe-medpro-government-contracts

49. Conn, D. (2022, January 11). Lords Watchdog Assesses Complaint Against Michelle Mone Over PPE Firm. *The Guardian*. https://www.theguardian.com/politics/2022/jan/11/lords-watchdog-assesses-complaint-against-michelle-mone-over-ppe-firm

50. Conn, D. (2022b, January 17). Lords Watchdog Launches Inquiry Into Michelle Mone Over 'VIP Lane' Contract. *The Guardian*. https://www.theguardian.com/politics/2022/jan/17/lords-standards-commissioner-launches-inquiry-into-michelle-mone

51. Emails between Lord Theodore Agnew and Michell Mone.

(2020, May 8). *The Guardian*. https://www.documentcloud.org/
documents/21469091-foi-response-private-emails-reveal-goves-role-in-
tory-linked-firms-ppe-contracts

52. Parliamentary Question response from Maggie Throup. UIN 81881,
tabled 25 November 2021 by Angela Rayner. (2022, February 17,).
UK Parliament. https://questions-statements.parliament.uk/written-
questions/detail/2021-11-25/81881

53. ICO Decision notice, reference: IC-149867-D8B9. (2023, May 25).
Information Commissioners Office. https://ico.org.uk/media/action-
weve-taken/decision-notices/2023/4025408/ic-149867-d8b9.pdf

54. Conn, D., Lewis, P., Dodd, V., & Rawlinson, K. (2022, April 29). Michelle
Mone's Home Raided As PPE Firm Linked To Tory Peer Investigated.
The Guardian. https://www.theguardian.com/uk-news/2022/apr/29/
nca-launches-investigation-ppe-firm-linked-to-michelle-mone

55. Dodd, V., Adu, A., & Conn, D. (2023, November 26). NCA Questions
Matt Hancock And Michael Gove In PPE Medpro Inquiry. *The
Guardian*. https://www.theguardian.com/uk-news/2023/nov/26/
matt-hancock-michael-gove-questioned-ppe-medpro-inquiry-national-
crime-agency

56. Conn, D. (2022c, November 23). Revealed: Tory Peer Michelle Mone
Secretly Received £29m From 'VIP Lane' PPE Firm. *The Guardian*.
https://www.theguardian.com/uk-news/2022/nov/23/revealed-tory-peer-
michelle-mone-secretly-received-29m-from-vip-lane-ppe-firm

57. Allegretti, A., & Elgot, J. (2022, December 6). Tory Peer Michelle Mone
To Take Leave Of Absence From House Of Lords. *The Guardian*. https://
www.theguardian.com/uk-news/2022/dec/06/tory-peer-michelle-mone-
to-take-leave-of-absence-from-house-of-lords

58. Particulars of Claim. The Secretary of State for Health and Social Care
and PPE Medpro Limited. High Court of Justice. (2022, December).
Financial Times. https://www.documentcloud.org/documents/23563617-
dhsc-v-ppe-medpro-particulars-of-claim

59. Howard Kennedy. (2023. February 27). PPE Medpro files defence
in High Court to £133 million UK Government lawsuit. https://
disputeresolution.howardkennedy.com/post/102i8p5/ppe-medpro-files-
defence-in-high-court-to-133-million-uk-government-lawsuit

60. Mark Williams-Thomas. Wikipedia Page. (2024, May 15). Wikipedia.
https://en.wikipedia.org/wiki/Mark_Williams-Thomas

61. Services – Specialist Investigations. (2024, May 15). Specialist
Investigations. https://specialistinvestigations.com/services/#media

62. Conn, D., & Scott, R. (2023, December 19). Revealed: Journalist Behind
Michelle Mone Film Also Worked As Private Investigator On Her

Notes

Behalf. *The Guardian.* https://www.theguardian.com/uk-news/2023/dec/19/revealed-journalist-behind-michelle-mone-film-also-worked-as-private-investigator-on-her-behalf

63. Covid Contracts: Dog Food Vendor Probably Earned £1m For PPE Deals. (2021, March 15). BBC News. https://www.bbc.co.uk/news/uk-56400527

64. Moss, V., & Drake, M. (2014, September 27). Tory Minister Brooks Newmark Quits Over Sex Scandal. *The Mirror.* https://www.mirror.co.uk/news/uk-news/tory-minister-brooks-newmark-quits-4335398

65. Pogrund, G., Greenwood, G., & Dyer, H. (2021, May 16). Matt Hancock Helped Tory Secure £180m PPE Deal. The Times. https://www.thetimes.co.uk/article/matt-hancock-helped-tory-secure-180m-ppe-deal-chv05lj3n

66. Supply Of Personal Protective Equipment For Healthcare Workers For The Care Of Patients With Suspected Or Confirmed Novel Coronavirus (COVID-19) – Contracts Finder. (2021, March 10). Contracts Finder. GOV.UK. https://www.contractsfinder.service.gov.uk/notice/44672d4a-7af2-4e38-a39a-edb06089f3c0?origin=SearchResults&p=1

67. Barr, L. (2022, February 6). Millions Of Safety Goggles Ordered For £178million Could Go To Waste. Mail Online. https://www.dailymail.co.uk/news/article-10481301/PPE-scandal-mounts-tens-millions-safety-goggles-ordered-178million-waste.html

68. Scott, R. (2023, January 24). REVEALED: Politically Connected Broker Made £17m Profit On 'VIP' PPE Contracts – Good Law Project. Good Law Project. https://goodlawproject.org/revealed-politically-connected-broker-made-17m-profit-on-vip-ppe-contracts/

69. Colbert, M. (2024, April 13), *Broker bought £7.25m manor house weeks after landing VIP lane contracts.* Good Law Project. https://goodlawproject.org/broker-bought-7-25m-manor-house-weeks-after-landing-vip-lane-contracts/

70. Summary Of Investigation – Brooks Newmark & Co Ltd – ORCL. (2024, February 13). Office of the Registrar of Consultant Lobbyists. https://registrarofconsultantlobbyists.org.uk/summary-of-investigation-brooks-newmark-co-ltd/

71. The loophole that enables secret lobbying by foreign companies (taxpolicy.org.uk) Neidle, D. (2024, February 16). The loophole that enables secret lobbying by foreign companies. Tax Policy. https://taxpolicy.org.uk/2024/02/16/lobbying/

72. Summary of investigation – The Rt. Hon. Owen Paterson. Published on: Wednesday 26th February 2025. Summary of investigation – The Rt. Hon. Owen Paterson – ORCL

73. The Electoral Commission. (2023, May 13). http://bit.ly/41gdope

74. Adams, R. (2018, January 24). David Meller, The Tory Donor 'desperate To Be Part Of Establishment.' *The Guardian*. https://www.theguardian.com/uk-news/2018/jan/24/david-meller-presidents-club-groping-scandal-wealthy-tory-donor

75. MELLER DESIGNS LIMITED Filing History – Find And Update Company Information – GOV.UK. (2024, May 15). Companies House. GOV.UK. https://find-and-update.company-information.service.gov.uk/company/00502663/filing-history

76. *Donor lobbied Michael Gove's office before fast-track PPE contract*. 2023, (June 26) The Times. https://www.thetimes.com/uk/politics/article/donor-lobbied-michael-goves-office-before-fast-track-ppe-contract-9gxwpbfrt

77. EXCLUSIVE: 4 More VIP-lane Companies Revealed – Good Law Project. (2021, April 29). Good Law Project. https://goodlawproject.org/update/awarded-contracts-vip-lane/?utm_source=Twitter&utm_medium=social%20media&utm_campaign=ppe%20hearing%202904

78. PPE Procurement In The Early Pandemic. (2021, November 17). GOV.UK. https://www.gov.uk/government/news/ppe-procurement-in-the-early-pandemic

79. MELLER DESIGNS LIMITED Filing History – Find And Update Company Information – GOV.UK. (2024, May 15). Companies House. GOV.UK. https://find-and-update.company-information.service.gov.uk/company/00502663/filing-history

80. VIP Lane Contracts Inflated By £925m – Good Law Project. (2023, December 11). Good Law Project. https://goodlawproject.org/vip-lane-contracts-inflated-by-925m/

81. Mason, R. (2023, December 10). PPE Bought Via 'VIP Lane' Was On Average 80% More Expensive, Documents Reveal. *The Guardian*. https://www.theguardian.com/world/2023/dec/10/ppe-via-vip-lane-average-80-percent-more-expensive-documents-reveal

82. Conn, D. (2024, February 20). Michael Gove Failed To Register Hospitality With Donor Whose Firm He Referred For PPE Contracts. *The Guardian*. https://www.theguardian.com/politics/2024/feb/20/michael-gove-failed-to-register-hospitality-from-donor-whose-firm-he-referred-for-ppe-contracts

83. Macken, L. (2022, November 26). Exclusive Brethren Family Pay $9.5 Million For Dural 'weekender.' The Sydney Morning Herald. https://www.smh.com.au/property/news/exclusive-brethren-family-pay-9-5-million-for-dural-weekender-20221124-p5c13h.html

84. Projects | Our Portfolio | Unispace. (2024, May 15). Unispace.Com.

https://www.unispace.com/projects?region=3

85. Scott, R. (2024, February 2). Michael Gove Opened The Door To Biggest VIP Lane Firm – Good Law Project. Good Law Project. https://goodlawproject.org/michael-gove-opened-the-door-to-biggest-vip-lane-firm/

86. Who Are The Brethren. (2024, May 15). OPEN & CANDID. https://www.openandcandid.com/who-are-the-brethren.html

87. Gray, C. (2023, February 24). Plymouth Brethren Christian Church: 'Cult' claims by Leeds man led family and friends to accuse him of harassment. Yorkshire Evening Post. https://www.yorkshireeveningpost.co.uk/news/crime/plymouth-brethren-christian-church-cult-claims-by-leeds-man-led-family-and-friends-to-accuse-him-of-harassment-3998334

88. Open & Candid, https://www.openandcandid.com/

89. Kenber, B., & Mostrous, A. (2015, March 17). Secretive Leader With Private Jet Is God's Man On Earth. The Times. https://www.thetimes.co.uk/article/secretive-leader-with-private-jet-is-gods-man-on-earth-zvcn72dgm7c

90. Kenber, B., & Mostrous, A. (n.d.). "No Mercy" – How A Tiny Christian Sect Made It To The Heart Of Westminster. The Times. Retrieved May 15, 2024, from https://times-deck.s3-eu-west-1.amazonaws.com/projects/470e7a4f017a5476afb7eeb3f8b96f9b.html

91. Scott, R. (2024, February 2). Michael Gove Opened The Door To Biggest VIP Lane Firm – Good Law Project. Good Law Project. https://goodlawproject.org/michael-gove-opened-the-door-to-biggest-vip-lane-firm/

92. Scott, R. (2024, February 2). Michael Gove Opened The Door To Biggest VIP Lane Firm – Good Law Project. Good Law Project. https://goodlawproject.org/michael-gove-opened-the-door-to-biggest-vip-lane-firm/

93. Parliamentary Question response from Edward Argar. UIN 118521, tabled04 February 2022 by Nick Smith. (2022, February 28,). UK Parliament. https://questions-statements.parliament.uk/written-questions/detail/2022-02-04/118521/

94. Hoyle, C. (2024, March 30). Exclusive Brethren Businesses Face Sweeping Tax Fraud Investigation. The Post. https://www.thepost.co.nz/nz-news/350230688/exclusive-brethren-businesses-face-sweeping-tax-fraud-investigation

95. PPE Procurement In The Early Pandemic. (2021b, November 17). GOV.UK. https://www.gov.uk/government/news/ppe-procurement-in-the-early-pandemic

96. Geoghegan, P., & Scott, R. (2020, November 13). Revealed:

Former Tory Chairman Was Secretly Appointed As COVID Advisor. OpenDemocracy. https://www.opendemocracy.net/en/dark-money-investigations/revealed-former-tory-chairman-was-secretly-appointed-covid-advisor/

97. Pickard, J. (2021, May 12). Former Tory Chair Faces Conflict Of Interest Claims Over PPE Contract. Financial Times. https://www.ft.com/content/b1659548-7cd0-4626-8406-7b2338d04489

98. Supply Of Personal Protective Equipment For Healthcare Workers For The Care Of Patients With Suspected Or Confirmed Novel Coronavirus (Covid-19) – Contracts Finder. (2021, March 8). Contracts Finder. GOV.UK. https://www.contractsfinder.service.gov.uk/notice/e4c5121f-5671-46fb-90c5-93a7e7c35f6a?origin=SearchResults&p=5

99. Geoghegan, P., & Scott, R. (2020, November 13). Revealed: Former Tory Chairman Was Secretly Appointed As COVID Advisor. OpenDemocracy. https://www.opendemocracy.net/en/dark-money-investigations/revealed-former-tory-chairman-was-secretly-appointed-covid-advisor/

100. Forrest, A. (2021, August 20). Labour Accuses Michael Gove Of Misleading Parliament Over £22m PPE Contract. The Independent. https://www.independent.co.uk/news/uk/politics/michael-gove-ppe-contract-labour-b1906025.html

101. Bunzl Healthcare: Protective Clothing. (2021, August 17). TheyWorkForYou. https://www.theyworkforyou.com/wrans/?id=2021-07-13.32410.h&s=bunzl

102. Management of PPE contracts Twelfth Report of Session 2022–23. (2022, July 20). House of Commons Committee of Public Accounts. https://committees.parliament.uk/publications/23109/documents/169286/default/

103. Kemp, P. (2020, November 18). Lord Feldman: Department Of Health Adviser's Firm Took Work From Covid Company. BBC News. https://www.bbc.co.uk/news/uk-54975507

104. Oxford Nanopore Technologies Ltd – Test Kits Assay, Reagents, Training Material And Support – Contracts Finder. (2020, May 18). Contracts Finder. GOV.UK. https://www.contractsfinder.service.gov.uk/notice/4cad12f6-cb34-4429-9e9c-e96c505ce9f5?origin=SearchResults&p=2

105. Oxford Nanopore Technologies Ltd – Provision Of LamPORE Testing Materials – Contracts Finder. (2020, November 6). Contracts Finder. GOV.UK. https://www.contractsfinder.service.gov.uk/notice/39876d00-f2ea-43ad-b521-4134bf897f7e?origin=SearchResults&p=2

106. OXFORD NANOPORE TECHNOLOGIES Plc Overview – Find

Notes

And Update Company Information – GOV.UK. (n.d.-b). Companies House. GOV.UK. Retrieved May 15, 2024, from https://find-and-update. company-information.service.gov.uk/company/05386273

107. PROMOVISE LIMITED Filing History – Find And Update Company Information – GOV.UK. (n.d.). Companies House. GOV.UK. Retrieved May 15, 2024, from https://find-and-update.company-information. service.gov.uk/company/09767522/filing-history

108. Lord Peter Chadlington donations to the Conservative Party registered. Electoral Commission website. Retrieved May 15, 2024, from http://bit. ly/3JkaARY

109. The conduct of Lord Chadlington. Commissioner Report 2023-24/6. House of Lords. Retrieved May 15, 2024, from https://www.parliament. uk/globalassets/documents/lords-commissioner-for-standards/conduct-of-lord-chadlington.pdf

110. Conn, D., & Evans, R. (2023, January 9). Conservative Peer Helped Land £50m PPE Contract For Firm Linked To Fellow Tory. *The Guardian.* https://www.theguardian.com/politics/2023/jan/09/conservative-peer-helped-land-50m-ppe-contract-for-firm-linked-to-fellow-tory

111. Supply Of Personal Protective Equipment For Healthcare Workers For The Care Of Patients With Suspected Or Confirmed Novel Coronavirus (Covid-19) – Contracts Finder. (2021b, March 18). Contracts Finder. GOV.UK. https://www.contractsfinder.service.gov.uk/notice/a9015913-35ef-44ad-bfc9-c0518aacaf2f?origin=SearchResults&p=1

112. Supply Of Personal Protective Equipment For Healthcare Workers For The Care Of Patients With Suspected Or Confirmed Novel Coronavirus (Covid-19) – Contracts Finder. (2020c, October 20). Contracts Finder. GOV.UK. https://www.contractsfinder.service.gov.uk/notice/2acda44b-6d22-424a-bd3d-ab539b50b967?origin=SearchResults&p=1

113. Half Of VIP Lane Companies Supplied PPE Worth £1 Billion That Was Not Fit For Purpose – Spotlight On Corruption. (2022, February 11). Spotlight On Corruption. https://www.spotlightcorruption.org/half-of-vip-lane-companies-supplied-ppe-worth-1-billion-that-was-not-fit-for-purpose/

114. Colbert, M. (2023, December 21). Firm Referred By Tory Peer Bagged PPE Contracts At Twice Average Price – Good Law Project. Good Law Project. https://goodlawproject.org/firm-referred-by-tory-peer-bagged-ppe-contracts-at-twice-average-price/

115. Conn, D., & Evans, R. (2023b, July 26). Government Likely To Lose Millions In Dispute Over PPE Contract Awarded Via 'VIP Lane.' *The Guardian.* https://www.theguardian.com/politics/2023/jul/26/government-millions-ppe-sg-recruitment-uk-lord-chadlington

116. PROMOVISE LIMITED Overview – Find And Update Company Information – GOV.UK. (n.d.). Companies House. GOV.UK. Retrieved May 15, 2024, from https://find-and-update.company-information. service.gov.uk/company/09767522

117. The conduct of Lord Chadlington. Commissioner Report 2023-24/6. House of Lords. Retrieved May 15, 2024, from https://www.parliament. uk/globalassets/documents/lords-commissioner-for-standards/conduct- of-lord-chadlington.pdf

118. Summary Of Investigation – Tulchan Communications LLP ('Tulchan') – ORCL. (2020, November 25). The Office of the Registrar of Consultant Lobbyists. https://registrarofconsultantlobbyists.org.uk/investigation- case-summary-tulchan-communications-llp-tulchan/

119. LUXE LIFESTYLE LIMITED Filing History – Find And Update Company Information – GOV.UK. (n.d.). Companies House. GOV. UK. Retrieved May 15, 2024, from https://find-and-update.company- information.service.gov.uk/company/11703750/filing-history

120. Supply Of Personal Protective Equipment For Healthcare Workers For The Care Of Patients With Suspected Or Confirmed Novel Coronavirus (Covid-19) – Contracts Finder. (2020a, June 23). Contracts Finder. GOV. UK. https://www.contractsfinder.service.gov.uk/notice/7e35428c-19bc- 4a2e-86fe-5e44def750d4?origin=SearchResults&p=1

121. Delahunty, S. (2020, July 2). Lifestyle Company With No Employees Or Trading History Handed £25 Million PPE Contract. *Byline Times.* https://bylinetimes.com/2020/07/02/lifestyle-company-with-no- employees-or-trading-history-handed-25-million-ppe-contract/

122. Lucas, C. (n.d.). Letter To Health Minister About PPE Contracts | Caroline Lucas. Carolinelucas.Com. Retrieved May 15, 2024, from https://www.carolinelucas.com/caroline/parliament/letter/letter-to- health-minister-about-ppe-contracts

123. Scott, Russell. (2021, April 29). *EXCLUSIVE: 4 more VIP-lane companies revealed.* Good Law Project. https://goodlawproject.org/update/awarded- contracts-vip-lane/

124. Half Of VIP Lane Companies Supplied PPE Worth £1 Billion That Was Not Fit For Purpose – Spotlight On Corruption. (2022b, February 11). Spotlight On Corruption. https://www.spotlightcorruption.org/ half-of-vip-lane-companies-supplied-ppe-worth-1-billion-that-was-not- fit-for-purpose/

125. LUXE LIFESTYLE LIMITED Filing History – Find And Update Company Information – GOV.UK. (n.d.). Companies House. GOV. UK. Retrieved May 15, 2024, from https://find-and-update.company- information.service.gov.uk/company/11703750/filing-history

Notes

126. Scott, R. (2023b, February 12). REVEALED: Greg Hands Referred Close Political Contact For £25m VIP Contract – Good Law Project. Good Law Project. https://goodlawproject.org/revealed-greg-hands-referred-close-political-contact-for-25m-vip-contract/

127. Mason, R. (2023a, February 12). Firm Won £25.8m PPE Contract After Greg Hands Approached By Tory Activist. *The Guardian*. https://www.theguardian.com/politics/2023/feb/12/firm-won-ppe-contract-greg-hands-approached-by-tory-activist-luxe-lifestyle

128. PPE Procurement In The Early Pandemic. (2021c, November 17). GOV.UK. http://web.archive.org/web/20211117181735/https://www.gov.uk/government/news/ppe-procurement-in-the-early-pandemic

129. Investigation Into Government Procurement During The Covid-19 Pandemic – NAO Press Release. (2020, November 26). National Audit Office (NAO). https://www.nao.org.uk/press-releases/government-procurement-during-the-covid-19-pandemic/

130. PPE Procurement In The Early Pandemic. (2021c, November 17). GOV.UK. http://web.archive.org/web/20211117181735/https://www.gov.uk/government/news/ppe-procurement-in-the-early-pandemic

131. Scott, R. (2022, February 8). Revealed: Ministers Have Misled Parliament About The Size Of The VIP Lane – Good Law Project. Good Law Project. https://goodlawproject.org/ministers-have-misled-parliament/

132. Ellery, B. (2022, February 14). Government Accused Of Cooking The Books On VIP Lane For Covid PPE Contracts. The Times. https://www.thetimes.co.uk/article/government-accused-of-cooking-the-books-on-vip-covid-contracts-qkd96vwzl

133. Supply Of Personal Protective Equipment For Healthcare Workers For The Care Of Patients With Suspected Or Confirmed Novel Coronavirus (Covid-19) – Contracts Finder. (2023, April 24). Contracts Finder. GOV.UK. https://www.contractsfinder.service.gov.uk/notice/ee49a66d-1532-4164-828b-57d1be9e6ac5?origin=SearchResults&p=1

134. BREAKING: Court Order Shows Boris Johnson Misled Parliament Over Covid Contracts – Good Law Project. (2021, March 5). Good Law Project. https://goodlawproject.org/update/johnson-misled-parliament/

135. Layton, J. (2021, March 8). Department Of Health Did £90,000,000 Deal With Firm Listed In Chinese Hotel Room. Metro. https://metro.co.uk/2021/03/08/hancocks-department-did-90m-ppe-deal-with-firm-listed-at-hotel-room-14210310/

136. Scott, R. (2022b, February 14). NEW: Leaked Emails Reveal Government Officials Manipulated VIP Lane Data After NAO Investigation – Good Law Project. Good Law Project. https://goodlawproject.org/leak-government-hid-vip-data/

137. Supply Of Personal Protective Equipment For Healthcare Workers For The Care Of Patients With Suspected Or Confirmed Novel Coronavirus (Covid-19) – Contracts Finder. (2020c, September 7). Contracts Finder. GOV.UK. https://www.contractsfinder.service.gov.uk/notice/c9fc3b9e-c1ca-470f-af06-559b6f9d67f9?origin=SearchResults&p=1

138. Scott, R. (2025, April 09). Woman Arrested in Fraud Investigation Linked to £25m 'VIP' Covid PPE Deal Referred by Conservative Minister. Byline Times. https://bylinetimes.com/2025/04/09/woman-arrested-in-fraud-investigation-linked-to-25m-vip-covid-ppe-deal-referred-by-conservative-minister/

139. Scott, R (2025, April 16). The Sheer Scale of the COVID 'VIP Lane' PPE Scandal Has Still Not Been Revealed Five Years On. Byline Times. https://bylinetimes.com/2025/04/16/covid-inquiry-vip-ppe/

140. Investigation into government procurement during the Covid-19 pandemic. (2020, November 26). National Audit Office. https://www.nao.org.uk/wp-content/uploads/2020/11/Investigation-into-government-procurement-during-the-Covid-19-pandemic.pdf

141. Scott, R. (2022b, February 14). NEW: Leaked Emails Reveal Government Officials Manipulated VIP Lane Data After NAO Investigation – Good Law Project. Good Law Project. https://goodlawproject.org/leak-government-hid-vip-data/

142. Scott, R. (2022b, February 14). NEW: Leaked Emails Reveal Government Officials Manipulated VIP Lane Data After NAO Investigation – Good Law Project. Good Law Project. https://goodlawproject.org/leak-government-hid-vip-data/

143. Hughes, D. (2024, February 6). Covid Inquiry To Look At Whether Some PPE Contracts Were 'fraudulent.' Evening Standard. https://www.standard.co.uk/news/politics/mps-national-audit-office-david-hughes-b1137410.html

Chapter 2: Test and Trace

1. Government Launches NHS Test And Trace Service. (2020, May 27). GOV.UK. https://www.gov.uk/government/news/government-launches-nhs-test-and-trace-service

2. £37 Billion Was The Two-year Budget For NHS Test And Trace, Not How Much Was Spent – Full Fact. (2022, May 16). Full Fact. https://fullfact.org/health/test-and-trace-37-billion/

3. 3 Scott, R. (2023, December 22). Lord Bethell's WhatsApp's With Matt Hancock And Dido Harding Released. https://russellscott.substack.com/p/lord-bethells-whatsapps-with-matt

4. Investigation into the government's contracts with Randox Laboratories

Ltd. (2022, March 24). National Audit Office. https://www.nao.org.uk/wp-content/uploads/2022/03/Investigation-into-the-governments-contracts-with-randox-laboratories-ltd.pdf

5. Scott, R. (2021, June 30). NEW: Documents Reveal VIP Lane For Testing Contracts – Good Law Project. Good Law Project. https://goodlawproject.org/vip-lane-for-testing-contracts/

6. Email dated 06/04/2020 Cairnduff To Minister's Offices. (n.d.). Good Law Project. Retrieved May 15, 2024, from https://drive.google.com/file/d/1tao6iPNNPitzIDM4xXdaf4jGIZq7-gLV/view

7. Conn, D. (2021, June 30). Concerns Over VIP Lane For Covid Testing Contracts After 'fast Track' Email Revealed. *The Guardian*. https://www.theguardian.com/politics/2021/jun/30/bids-from-politically-connected-firms-for-covid-test-contracts-designated-fast-track-email-suggests

8. Conn, D. (2021, July 15). Firm with ties to Hancock given 'VIP treatment', emails suggest. The Guardian. Firm with ties to Hancock given 'VIP treatment', emails suggest | Coronavirus | The Guardian

9. Lateral Flow Test Kits – Contracts Finder. (2020, December 11). Contracts Finder. GOV.UK. https://www.contractsfinder.service.gov.uk/notice/c4be5045-2dc2-43b7-9de2-7b691832952a?origin=SearchResults&p=1

10. Scott, R. (2021b, September 23). BREAKING: Government Misled Public Over Existence Of VIP Lane For Testing Contracts – Good Law Project. Good Law Project. https://goodlawproject.org/update/breaking-government-misled-public-over-existence-of-vip-lane-for-testing-contracts/

11. Covid-19 Contracts: High Priority Lane. (2022, February 24). TheyWorkForYou. https://www.theyworkforyou.com/debates/?id=2022-02-24c.448.6&s=%22high+priority+lane%22

12. ICO Decision Notice. Reference IC-150101-Z2Z4. (2022, November 3). Good Law Project. https://drive.google.com/file/d/1Jp1p_b_8q0qXwGVkvcFeaGWj9wR0-anJ/view

13. Scott, R. (2022, December 21). REVEALED: The Names Of Those Who Referred Covid Testing Firms Into The "VIP" Lane – Good Law Project. Good Law Project. https://goodlawproject.org/revealed-the-names-of-those-who-referred-covid-testing-firms-into-the-vip-lane/

14. UK Health Security Agency FOI response reference 03/11/22/KMG/1000, Referrers to the Covid testing 'VIP' route. (2022, December 21). Good Law Project. https://drive.google.com/file/d/1i1DhMGaIvuQlfqn2tTUiBC0TcNy5rYll/view

15. Investigation into the government's contracts with Randox Laboratories Ltd. (2022, March 24). National Audit Office. https://www.nao.org.

uk/wp-content/uploads/2022/03/Investigation-into-the-governments-contracts-with-randox-laboratories-ltd.pdf

16. Brooks, R. (n.d.). Profits of Doom. Private Eye. Retrieved May 15, 2024, from https://www.private-eye.co.uk/pictures/special_reports/profits-of-doom.pdf

17. – Executives. (n.d.). Pasaca Capital. Retrieved May 15, 2024, from https://pasacacapital.com/executives/

18. Darmiento, L., Peterson, M., & Flemming, J. (2021, July 28). A Pasadena Startup Got Billions Selling Covid Tests. Then Came Questions. Los Angeles Times. https://www.latimes.com/business/story/2021-07-28/innova-pasaca-covid-17-antigen-test-british-uk-government

19. Boseley, S., & Lawrence, F. (2021, January 28). How UK Spent £800m On Controversial Covid Tests For Dominic Cummings Scheme. *The Guardian*. https://www.theguardian.com/world/2021/jan/28/how-uk-spent-800m-on-controversial-covid-tests-for-dominic-cummings-scheme

20. SARS-CoV-2 Antigen Rapid Qualitative Test Kits – Contracts Finder. (2020, December 2). Contracts Finder. GOV.UK. https://www.contractsfinder.service.gov.uk/notice/ca07d68e-8f93-4864-9c4b-f24f1e117162?origin=SearchResults&p=1

21. Contracts Finder. GOV.UK. Retrieved May 15, 2024, from https://www.contractsfinder.service.gov.uk/Search/Results?page=1#ca07d68e-8f93-4864-9c4b-f24f1e117162

22. Stop Using Innova SARS-CoV-2 Antigen Rapid Qualitative Test. (2021, June 10). US Food And Drug Administration. https://web.archive.org/web/20210618185400/https://www.fda.gov/medical-devices/safety-communications/stop-using-innova-sars-cov-2-antigen-rapid-qualitative-test-fda-safety-communication

23. Warning Letter, Innova Medical Group, Inc. MARCS-CMS 614819 (2021, June 10). US Food & Drug Administration. https://www.fda.gov/inspections-compliance-enforcement-and-criminal-investigations/warning-letters/innova-medical-group-inc-614819-06102021

24. Stop Using Innova SARS-CoV-2 Antigen Rapid Qualitative Test. (2021, June 10). US Food And Drug Administration. https://web.archive.org/web/20210618185400/https://www.fda.gov/medical-devices/safety-communications/stop-using-innova-sars-cov-2-antigen-rapid-qualitative-test-fda-safety-communication

25. Boseley, S., & Lawrence, F. (2021, January 28). How UK Spent £800m On Controversial Covid Tests For Dominic Cummings Scheme. *The Guardian*. https://www.theguardian.com/world/2021/jan/28/how-uk-spent-800m-on-controversial-covid-tests-for-dominic-cummings-scheme

26. Provision Of Lateral Flow Testing Devices – Contracts Finder. (2021,

November 24). Contracts Finder. GOV.UK. https://www.contractsfinder.
service.gov.uk/notice/8ae569d0-5ab7-41d0-a900-7d95497feac1?origin=S
earchResults&p=1

27. Scott, R. (2022b, December 21). REVEALED: The Names Of Those
Who Referred Covid Testing Firms Into The "VIP" Lane – Good Law
Project. Good Law Project. https://goodlawproject.org/revealed-the-
names-of-those-who-referred-covid-testing-firms-into-the-vip-lane/

28. UK Health Security Agency FOI response reference 03/11/22/
KMG/1000, Referrers to the Covid testing 'VIP' route. (2022, December
21). Good Law Project. https://drive.google.com/file/d/1i1DhMGaIvuQl
fqn2tTUiBC0TcNy5rYll/view

29. Emma Stanton LinkedIn Profile. Retrieved May 15, 2024, from https://
www.linkedin.com/in/emmastanton/?originalSubdomain=uk

30. Our Senior Team. (n.d.). BioNTech. Retrieved May 15, 2024, from
https://www.BioNTech.com/int/en/home/about/our-senior-team.html

31. Scott, R. (2023a, February 24). Revealed: Company With Just
£85 In The Bank Made £20m Profit After Dominic Cummings
Referred Innova Medical Into The 'VIP' Lane – Good Law
Project. Good Law Project. https://goodlawproject.org/
new-company-with-just-85-in-the-bank-made-20m-profit-after-
dominic-cummings-referred-innova-medical-into-the-vip-lane/

32. Email from Kim Thonger to Dominic Cummings dated 29 July 2020.
(n.d.). Good Law Project. Retrieved May 15, 2024, from https://drive.
google.com/file/d/1iss3u9uIlaY9veAC6FCgj4psch1r7ePG/view

33. Cummings, D. (2023, October 12). INQ000273872 – Witness Statement
Of Dominic Cummings Dated 12/10/2023. UK Covid-19 Inquiry
Archives. UK Covid-19 Inquiry. https://covid19.public-inquiry.uk/
documents/inq000273872-witness-statement-of-dominic-cummings-
dated-12-10-2023/

34. Scott, R. (2023a, February 24). Revealed: Company With Just
£85 In The Bank Made £20m Profit After Dominic Cummings
Referred Innova Medical Into The 'VIP' Lane – Good Law
Project. Good Law Project. https://goodlawproject.org/
new-company-with-just-85-in-the-bank-made-20m-profit-after-
dominic-cummings-referred-innova-medical-into-the-vip-lane/

35. DISRUPTIVE NANOTECHNOLOGY LIMITED Filing History –
Find And Update Company Information – GOV.UK. (n.d.). Companies
House. GOV.UK. Retrieved May 16, 2024, from https://find-and-update.
company-information.service.gov.uk/company/09331606/filing-history

36. Darmiento, L., Peterson, M., & Flemming, J. (2021, July 28). A Pasadena
Startup Got Billions Selling Covid Tests. Then Came Questions. Los

Angeles Times. https://www.latimes.com/business/story/2021-07-28/
innova-pasaca-covid-17-antigen-test-british-uk-government

37. Grateful Ex-student Donates £50m To Strathclyde University. (2021,
September 21). BBC News. https://www.bbc.co.uk/news/uk-scotland-
glasgow-west-58628270

38. Conn, D. Scott, R. (2024, June 17). Boss of US firm given £4bn in UK
Covid contracts accused of squandering millions on jets and properties.
The Guardian. https://www.theguardian.com/world/article/2024/jun/17/
boss-us-firm-uk-covid-contracts-accused-squandering-millions-on-jets-
properties

39. Geoghegan, P. Scott, R. (2024, September 26). Exclusive: Tony Blair
advising Covid contract 'overnight billionaire'. Democracy for Sale.
https://democracyforsale.substack.com/p/exclusive-tony-blair-advising-
covid

40. Scott, R. (2023b, March 13). £250m Wasted On 'VIP' Covid Tests
– Good Law Project. Good Law Project. https://goodlawproject.
org/250m-wasted-on-vip-covid-tests/

41. E-Auction (Online Asset Disposal) Services – Contracts Finder. (2023,
April 12). Contracts Finder. GOV.UK. https://www.contractsfinder.
service.gov.uk/notice/c0e4265f-9c11-476b-a0c4-d6b0be75a006?origin=S
earchResults&p=1

42. Covid 19 Rapid Antigen Test Self-Test Kit – Lot No.X2104005 – 23
Boxes (56 Packs Of 7 Per Box). (n.d.). AUCTIONS.RAMCO.UK.
Retrieved May 16, 2024, from https://auctions.ramco.uk/past-auctions/
ramco-11335/lot-details/bc538df2-9419-4136-ba6d-b0dc0100d531

43. Contract For Reimbursement Of Manufacturing Costs With Option To
Purchase Goods – Contracts Finder. (2021, January 22). Contracts Finder.
GOV.UK. https://www.contractsfinder.service.gov.uk/notice/5cbbec8c-
bef2-4e29-9c9e-9f4921a8eb79?origin=SearchResults&p=1

44. Contract For The Supply Of Raw Materials For Manufacture Of Lateral
Flow Tests – Contracts Finder. (2021, March 23). Contracts Finder.
GOV.UK. https://www.contractsfinder.service.gov.uk/notice/c8c27e87-
6340-4917-8320-dd0ab41f5864?origin=SearchResults&p=1

45. 45 Manufacture Of Lateral Flow Antigen Tests For SARS-CoV-2 –
Contracts Finder. (2021, February 17). Contracts Finder. GOV.UK.
https://www.contractsfinder.service.gov.uk/notice/8339319b-b512-4820-
a1e0-48bf8561ac3a?origin=SearchResults&p=1

46. 46 British Manufacturer SureScreen Diagnostics To Supply 20 Million
Rapid Lateral Flow. (2021, February 8). GOV.UK. https://www.gov.
uk/government/news/british-manufacturer-SureScreen-diagnostics-to-
supply-20-million-rapid-lateral-flow

Notes

47. SURESCREEN HOLDINGS LIMITED Filing History – Find And Update Company Information – GOV.UK. (n.d.). Companies House. GOV.UK. Retrieved May 16, 2024, from https://find-and-update. company-information.service.gov.uk/company/09067025/filing-history

48. SURESCREEN HOLDINGS LIMITED Filing History – Find And Update Company Information – GOV.UK. (n.d.). Companies House. GOV.UK. Retrieved May 16, 2024, from https://find-and-update. company-information.service.gov.uk/company/09067025/filing-history

49. Emails Reveal Another VIP Test And Trace Contract That Leads To More Questions Than Answers – Good Law Project. (2022, September 3). Good Law Project. https://goodlawproject.org/vip-test-and-trace-SureScreen/

50. Scott, R. (2022c, December 21). REVEALED: The Names Of Those Who Referred Covid Testing Firms Into The "VIP" Lane – Good Law Project. Good Law Project. https://goodlawproject.org/revealed-the-names-of-those-who-referred-covid-testing-firms-into-the-vip-lane/

51. View Donation – The Electoral Commission. SureScreen Diagnostics Ltd donation to The Rt Hon Dr Liam Fox MP. (n.d.). The Electoral Commission. Retrieved May 16, 2024, from https://search. electoralcommission.org.uk/English/Donations/C0559762

52. REGISTER OF MEMBERS' FINANCIAL INTERESTS updates 12 July – 8 August 2022. UK Parliament. Retrieved May 16, 2024, from https://publications.parliament.uk/pa/cm/cmregmem/220808/ Updates%20-%2012%20July%20-%208%20August%202022.pdf

53. Kemp, P. (2022, September 3). Ex-minister Liam Fox Gets Donation From Covid Test Firm He Recommended. BBC News. https://www.bbc. co.uk/news/uk-politics-62766148

54. Clinton, J., & Cooney, C. (2022, September 4). MP Liam Fox Dismisses Reports About Donation From Covid Firm As 'baseless Smear.' *The Guardian*. https://www.theguardian.com/uk-news/2022/sep/04/mp-liam-fox-dismisses-reports-about-donation-from-covid-firm-as-baseless-smear

55. Close Friend Of MP Involved With Company Handed A Multi-million Covid Testing Contract – Good Law Project. (2022, October 13). Good Law Project. https://goodlawproject.org/SureScreenupdate131022/

56. Adam Werritty: Fox's Friend, Flatmate And Business Partner. (2011, October 14). BBC News. https://www.bbc.co.uk/news/uk-politics-15238289

57. Adam Werritty: Fox's Friend, Flatmate And Business Partner. (2011, October 14). BBC News. https://www.bbc.co.uk/news/uk-politics-15238289

58. Liam Fox Resignation Letters In Full. (2011, October 14). BBC News.

https://www.bbc.co.uk/news/uk-15311615

59. 2022.10.06[redacted] TW Letter To The Good Law Project.pdf. (n.d.). Good Law Project. Retrieved May 16, 2024, from https://drive.google. com/file/d/1KjEdezIkKeYo1F-rwCIP9dZAX8ztkdUl/view

60. Provision Of End-to-end Serology Testing Service For Covid-19 Testing – Contracts Finder. (2021, January 15). Contracts Finder. GOV.UK. https://www.contractsfinder.service.gov.uk/notice/49083f42-3699-4098-afab-5817507a1423?origin=SearchResults&p=1

61. Transparency data DHSC: ministerial gifts, hospitality, travel and meetings, April to June 2020. (2020, October 29). Gov.Uk. https://www.google.com/url?q=https://www.gov.uk/government/publications/dhsc-ministerial-gifts-hospitality-travel-and-meetings-april-to-june-2020&sa=D&source=docs&ust=1715897385721689&usg=AOvVaw0UBZhNUnWwwetubYp9hI2P

62. Home Antibody Testing Service – Contracts Finder. (2021, July 22). Contracts Finder. GOV.UK. https://www.contractsfinder.service.gov.uk/notice/428d6de8-3043-4e17-a226-be36aaafdb68?origin=SearchResults&p=1

63. National Microbiology Framework – Lot four Clinical Laboratory Diagnostic Testing Services – Contracts Finder. (2021, April 19). Contracts Finder. GOV.UK. https://www.contractsfinder.service.gov.uk/notice/bb6dfad6-f6e9-48ee-bb1f-3d93f307b451?origin=SearchResults&p=1

64. THRIVA LIMITED Filing History – Find And Update Company Information – GOV.UK. (n.d.). Companies House. GOV.UK. Retrieved May 16, 2024, from https://find-and-update.company-information.service.gov.uk/company/09828160/filing-history

65. Jonathan Djanogly Non-Executive Chairman Profile. (n.d.). Pembroke VCT. Retrieved May 16, 2024, from https://www.pembrokevct.com/our_people/jonathan-djanogly/

66. Rose, D. (2021, November 12). Jonathan Djanogly MP 'paid Nearly £1,000 An Hour By Firm.' Mail Online. https://www.dailymail.co.uk/news/article-10196915/Jonathan-Djanogly-MP-paid-nearly-1-000-hour-firm-benefits-NHS-Covid-contracts.html

67. Andrew Wolfson CEO Profile. (n.d.). Pembroke VCT. Retrieved May 16, 2024, from https://www.pembrokevct.com/our_people/andrew-wolfson/

68. REGISTER OF LORDS' INTERESTS. House of Lords. Retrieved May 16, 2024, from https://www.parliament.uk/globalassets/documents/publications-records/house-of-lords-publications/records-activities-and-membership/register-of-lords-interests/register180423.pdf

69. Baroness Blackwood profile. (n.d.). GOV.UK. Retrieved May 16, 2024,

from https://www.gov.uk/government/people/nicola-blackwood

70. Register of Interests – Members of the House of Lords. House. Baroness Blackwood of North Oxford. House of Lords. Retrieved May 16, 2024, from https://members.parliament.uk/members/lords/interests/register-of-lords-interests?SearchTerm=thriva&ShowAmendments=False

71. Meet our Advisory Board. (n.d.). Thriva. Retrieved May 16, 2024, from https://thrivasolutions.com/advisors

72. Thriva Appoints New Advisory Board. (2023, February 6). Thriva. https://thrivasolutions.com/thriva-appoints-new-advisory-board

73. Stewart, H. (2020, November 15). Labour Criticises Lobbyist's Involvement In Covid Strategy Calls. *The Guardian*. https://www.theguardian.com/politics/2020/nov/15/labour-criticises-lobbyists-involvement-in-covid-strategy-calls

74. Hickman, A. (2020, November 30). PRCA Probe Into Portland Dropped Following Lord O'Shaughnessy Exit. PR Week. https://www.prweek.com/article/1701384/prca-probe-portland-dropped-following-lord-oshaughnessy-exit

75. UK Health Security Agency FOI response reference 03/11/22/KMG/1000, Referrers to the Covid testing 'VIP' routed. (2022, December 21). Good Law Project. https://drive.google.com/file/d/1i1DhMGaIvuQlfqn2tTUiBC0TcNy5rYll/view

76. PCR Testing Services – Contracts Finder. (2020, December 1). Contracts Finder. GOV.UK. https://www.contractsfinder.service.gov.uk/notice/b6081829-dff9-4b7e-a483-de8564593563?origin=SearchResults&p=1

77. Final report of the Serious Untoward Incident investigation into the misreporting of PCR test results by the Immensa Health Clinic Limited. (2022, November). UK Health Security Agency. https://assets.publishing.service.gov.uk/government/uploads/system/uploads/attachment_data/file/1128035/SUI_INVESTIGATION_FINAL_REPORT.pdf

78. Crowson, I., James, E., & Ridley, S. (2021, January 31). Workers At Covid Testing Centre Shown 'fighting & Boozing' In Shocking Video. The Sun. https://www.thesun.co.uk/news/13900590/workers-covid-testing-centre-fight-booze/

79. Final report of the Serious Untoward Incident investigation into the misreporting of PCR test results by the Immensa Health Clinic Limited. (2022, November). UK Health Security Agency. https://assets.publishing.service.gov.uk/government/uploads/system/uploads/attachment_data/file/1128035/SUI_INVESTIGATION_FINAL_REPORT.pdf

80. Services Provided For Laboratory Testing Services Of Covid-19 Samples – Contracts Finder. (2022, November 16). Contracts Finder. GOV.UK. https://www.contractsfinder.service.gov.uk/notice/dd2b4c9a-387f-4662-

a915-6e7a1ae2598f?origin=SearchResults&p=1

81. Final report of the Serious Untoward Incident investigation into the misreporting of PCR test results by the Immensa Health Clinic Limited. (2022, November). UK Health Security Agency. https://assets.publishing. service.gov.uk/government/uploads/system/uploads/attachment_data/ file/1128035/SUI_INVESTIGATION_FINAL_REPORT.pdf

82. Hill, M. (2022, November 29). Immensa Lab Errors May Have Led To 23 Covid-19 Deaths. BBC News. https://www.bbc.co.uk/news/ uk-england-63795285

83. Scott, R. (2022c, December 21). REVEALED: The Names Of Those Who Referred Covid Testing Firms Into The "VIP" Lane – Good Law Project. Good Law Project. https://goodlawproject.org/revealed-the-names-of-those-who-referred-covid-testing-firms-into-the-vip-lane/

84. Scott, R. (2022c, December 21). REVEALED: The Names Of Those Who Referred Covid Testing Firms Into The "VIP" Lane – Good Law Project. Good Law Project. https://goodlawproject.org/revealed-the-names-of-those-who-referred-covid-testing-firms-into-the-vip-lane/

85. Abbott In The UK | Abbott UK. (n.d.). Abbott. Retrieved May 16, 2024, from https://www.abbott.co.uk/about-abbott/abbott-in-the-uk.html

86. Serology – Rapid Antibody Test Kits – Contracts Finder. (2021, February 2). Contracts Finder. GOV.UK. https://www.contractsfinder.service.gov. uk/notice/e30710b0-d095-4431-8448-8fdb1e82654c?origin=SearchRes ults&p=1

87. Abbott Quotation reference Q2C-41932. (n.d.). Contracts Finder. GOV.UK. Retrieved May 16, 2024, from https://atamis-1928. my.salesforce.com/sfc/p/#0O000000rwim/a/4J000000kFuG/ J3Twc10jo5eT0GyjpjvRycGhsMmIF_FSO5NzYwSx1oY

88. Open Access UK: Monitor Lobbying Meetings With Government. (n.d.). Openaccess.Transparency.Org.Uk. Retrieved May 16, 2024, from https:// openaccess.transparency.org.uk/?meeting=62543

89. Open Access UK: Monitor Lobbying Meetings With Government. (n.d.-b). Https://Openaccess.Transparency.Org.Uk/. Retrieved May 16, 2024, from https://openaccess.transparency.org.uk/?meeting=64473

90. 90.Abbott Department of Health and Social Care written question – answered at on 22 March 2022. (2022, March 22). TheyWorkForYou. https://www.theyworkforyou.com/wrans/?id=2022-01-13.103702.h&s=ab bott+feldman#g103702.q0

91. Provision Of Abbott Panbio Covid 19 Antigen Rapid Test Devices – Contracts Finder. (2020, November 24). Contracts Finder. GOV.UK. https://www.contractsfinder.service.gov.uk/notice/80a130f3-fbfa-4134-9911-637d79c19c28?origin=SearchResults&p=1

92. Panbio Covid 19 Antigen Rapid Test - Contracts Finder (2020, November 27). https://www.contractsfinder.service.gov.uk/notice/ f4813108-a7e7-4485-8ce4-de3128daf27f?origin=SearchResults&p=1

93. UK Health Security Agency FOI response reference 03/11/22/ KMG/1000, Referrers to the Covid testing 'VIP' routed. (2022, December 21). Good Law Project. https://drive.google.com/file/d/1i1DhMGaIvuQl fqn2tTUiBC0TcNy5rYll/view

94. NATIONWIDE PATHOLOGY LIMITED Filing History – Find And Update Company Information – GOV.UK. (n.d.). Companies House. GOV.UK. Retrieved May 16, 2024, from https://find-and-update. company-information.service.gov.uk/company/07427189/filing-history

95. Planning Application – WND/2023/0018. (n.d.). West Northamptonshire Council. Retrieved May 16, 2024, from https://wnc. planning-register.co.uk/Planning/Display/WND/2023/0018

96. Planning Application – 2023/5312/FULL Skip. (n.d.). West Northamptonshire Council. Retrieved May 16, 2024, from https://wnc. planning-register.co.uk/Planning/Display/2023/5312/FULL#undefined

97. Covid-19 Testing Procurement. (2022, December 21). UK Health Security Agency. https://www.gov.uk/government/publications/covid-19-testing-procurement/covid-19-testing-procuremen

98. Investigation into the government's contracts with Randox Laboratories Ltd. (2022, March 24). National Audit Office. https://www.nao.org. uk/wp-content/uploads/2022/03/Investigation-into-the-governments-contracts-with-randox-laboratories-ltd.pdf

99. Randox Laboratories – Contract For The Delivery Of Covid-19 Testing; – Contracts Finder. (2020, May 18). Contracts Finder. GOV.UK. https:// www.contractsfinder.service.gov.uk/notice/7f989fa6-30e6-4caa-b28f-2b98fcce21c4?origin=SearchResults&p=1

100.Qnostics | Molecular Infectious Disease Controls | Randox. (n.d.). Randox Laboratories. Retrieved May 16, 2024, from https://www.randox. com/molecular-infectious-disease-controls/

101.RANDOX LABORATORIES LIMITED Filing History – Find And Update Company Information – GOV.UK. (n.d.). Companies House. GOV.UK. Retrieved May 16, 2024, from https://find-and-update. company-information.service.gov.uk/company/NI015738/filing-history

102.QNOSTICS LIMITED People – Find And Update Company Information – GOV.UK. (n.d.). Companies House. GOV.UK. Retrieved May 16, 2024, from https://find-and-update.company-information. service.gov.uk/company/SC257629/officers

103.Treasury Minutes Government Response to the Committee of Public Accounts on the Eleventh, Twelfth and Seventeenth reports from Session

2022-23. (2022, November). HM Treasury. https://assets.publishing. service.gov.uk/media/6368d7498fa8f57a1bd79f56/E02819805_CP_755_ TM_Gov_Resp_to_PAC_11_12_17_Accessible.pdf

104.Return to an Address of the Honourable the House of Commons dated 17 November 2021 for specified minutes, notes, and correspondence relating to Government contracts awarded to Randox Laboratories Ltd. (n.d.). House of Commons. Retrieved May 16, 2024, from https:// assets.publishing.service.gov.uk/media/61fc14c5e90e0768aabbde44/ government-response-to-humble-address-motion-on-randox-contracts. pdf

105.Investigation into the government's contracts with Randox Laboratories Ltd. (2022, March 24). National Audit Office. https://www.nao.org. uk/wp-content/uploads/2022/03/Investigation-into-the-governments-contracts-with-randox-laboratories-ltd.pdf

106.Evans, R., Lawrence, F., & Pegg, D. (2019, September 30). Revealed: Owen Paterson Lobbied For Firms He Was Paid To Advise. *The Guardian.* https://www.theguardian.com/politics/2019/sep/30/revealed-owen-paterson-lobbied-for-firms-he-was-paid-to-advise

107.Investigation into the government's contracts with Randox Laboratories Ltd. (2022, March 24). National Audit Office. https://www.nao.org. uk/wp-content/uploads/2022/03/Investigation-into-the-governments-contracts-with-randox-laboratories-ltd.pdf

108.Allegretti, A. (2021, October 26). MP Owen Paterson Faces Suspension For Breaking Lobbying Rules. *The Guardian.* https://www.theguardian. com/politics/2021/oct/26/owen-paterson-faces-suspension-breaking-lobbying-rules#:~:text=The%20committee%20revealed%20Paterson%20 had,%2Dfunded%20Commons%2Dheaded%20notepaper.

109.Randox Laboratories Ltd donations to political parties. The Electoral Commission. Retrieved May 16, 2024, from http://bit.ly/3JoC09j

110.Return to an Address of the Honourable the House of Commons dated 17 November 2021 for specified minutes, notes, and correspondence relating to Government contracts awarded to Randox Laboratories Ltd. (n.d.). House of Commons. Retrieved May 16, 2024, from https:// assets.publishing.service.gov.uk/media/61fc14c5e90e0768aabbde44/ government-response-to-humble-address-motion-on-randox-contracts. pdf

111.Investigation into the government's contracts with Randox Laboratories Ltd. (2022, March 24). National Audit Office. https://www.nao.org. uk/wp-content/uploads/2022/03/Investigation-into-the-governments-contracts-with-randox-laboratories-ltd.pdf

112.Randox Laboratories – Contract For The Delivery Of Covid-19 Testing;

– Contracts Finder. (2020b, May 18). Contracts Finder. GOV.UK. https://www.contractsfinder.service.gov.uk/notice/7f989fa6-30e6-4caa-b28f-2b98fcce21c4?origin=SearchResults&p=1

113. Update On Randox Test Kits. (2020, August 7). GOV.UK. https://www.gov.uk/government/news/update-on-randox-test-kits--2

114. Busby, M. (2020, August 8). Up To 750,000 UK Covid Test Kits Recalled Due To Safety Concerns. *The Guardian.* https://www.theguardian.com/world/2020/aug/08/up-to-750000-uk-randox-covid-test-kits-recalled-over-safety-concerns

115. Randox Laboratories Ltd Testing Services – Contracts Finder. (2020, November 26). Contracts Finder. GOV.UK. https://www.contractsfinder.service.gov.uk/notice/77691c09-d5fa-4093-8f18-1344f8a2c91b?origin=SearchResults&p=1

116. Investigation into the government's contracts with Randox Laboratories Ltd. (2022, March 24). National Audit Office. https://www.nao.org.uk/wp-content/uploads/2022/03/Investigation-into-the-governments-contracts-with-randox-laboratories-ltd.pdf

117. Return to an Address of the Honourable the House of Commons dated 17 November 2021 for specified minutes, notes, and correspondence relating to Government contracts awarded to Randox Laboratories Ltd. (n.d.). House of Commons. Retrieved May 16, 2024, from https://assets.publishing.service.gov.uk/media/61fc14c5e90e0768aabbde44/government-response-to-humble-address-motion-on-randox-contracts.pdf

118. Dispatches Investigation Into Covid Testing Firm Randox Sparked Major Health And Safety Probe | Channel 4. (2022, March 24). Channel 4 Dispatches. https://www.channel4.com/press/news/dispatches-investigation-covid-testing-firm-randox-sparked-major-health-and-safety-probe

119. Investigation into the government's contracts with Randox Laboratories Ltd. (2022, March 24). National Audit Office. https://www.nao.org.uk/wp-content/uploads/2022/03/Investigation-into-the-governments-contracts-with-randox-laboratories-ltd.pdf

120. RANDOX HOLDINGS LIMITED Filing History – Find And Update Company Information – GOV.UK. (n.d.). Companies House. GOV.UK. Retrieved May 16, 2024, from https://find-and-update.company-information.service.gov.uk/company/NI614690/filing-history

121. 121. Campbell, J. (2022, June 25). Randox Made Pre-tax Profit Of £275m In 2021. BBC News. https://www.bbc.co.uk/news/uk-northern-ireland-61935146

122. Campbell, J. (2023, June 28). Randox Made Pre-tax Profits Of £190m

In 2022, Accounts Show. BBC News. https://www.bbc.co.uk/news/uk-northern-ireland-66042684#:~:text=Randox%2C%20a%20major%20provider%20of,the%20government%27s%20National%20Testing%20Programme.

123. Hardman, I. (2021, November 17). Boris Johnson Shows His Lack Of Grip. The Spectator. https://www.spectator.co.uk/article/boris-johnson-shows-his-lack-of-grip/

124. Morris, S. (2021, November 17). Owen Paterson: Minister Confirms Government 'unable To Locate' Minutes Of Call Between Ex-Tory MP, Randox And Officials. Sky News. https://news.sky.com/story/owen-paterson-minister-confirms-government-unable-to-locate-minutes-of-meeting-between-ex-tory-mp-randox-and-officials-12470899

125. Committee on Standards publish report on the conduct of Rt Hon Owen Paterson MP (2021, October 26). UK Parliament. https://committees.parliament.uk/committee/290/committee-on-standards/news/158246/committee-on-standards-publish-report-on-the-conduct-of-rt-hon-owen-paterson-mp/

126. Government's contracts with Randox Laboratories Ltd Seventeenth Report of Session 2022–23. (2002, July 20). House of Commons. https://committees.parliament.uk/publications/23257/documents/169721/default/

127. Committee of Public Accounts. Randox Laboratories Ltd donations to political parties. The Electoral Commission. Retrieved May 16, 2024, from http://bit.ly/4mrZVDa

128. Test and Trace update Twenty-Third Report of Session 2021–22. (2021, October 21). House of Commons Committee of Public Accounts. https://committees.parliament.uk/publications/7651/documents/79945/default/

129. Scott, R. (2023, October 18). US banker paid himself £149m in dividends from lucrative UK government Covid testing deals. Torchlight: Russell Scott's Substack. https://russellscott.substack.com/p/us-banker-paid-himself-149m-in-dividends

130. TANNER PHARMA UK LIMITED Filing History – Find And Update Company Information – GOV.UK. (n.d.). Companies House. OV.UK. Retrieved January 07, 2025, from https://find-and-update.company-information.service.gov.uk/company/09566234/filing-history

Chapter 3: The peers

1. Lord James Bethell political donations. The Electoral Commission. Retrieved May 16, 2024, from http://bit.ly/41fp3Vj

2. NQ000237819 – Witness Statement Of Lord Udny-Lister, Former Downing Street Chief Of Staff, Dated 09/08/2023. UK Covid-19 Inquiry Archives. (2023, November 7). UK Covid-19 Inquiry. https://covid19.

public-inquiry.uk/documents/inq000237819-witness-statement-of-lord-udny-lister-former-downing-street-chief-of-staff-dated-09-08-2023/

3. Lord Deighton profile. (n.d.). GOV.UK. Retrieved May 16, 2024, from https://www.gov.uk/government/people/paul-deighton

4. Bradley, J., Gebrekidan, S., & McCann, A. (2020, December 17). Waste, Negligence And Cronyism: Inside Britain's Pandemic Spending (Published 2020). The New York Times. https://www.nytimes.com/interactive/2020/12/17/world/europe/britain-covid-contracts.html

5. Supply Of Personal Protective Equipment For Healthcare Workers For The Care Of Patients With Suspected Or Confirmed Novel Coronavirus (Covid-19) – Contracts Finder. (2020, June 23). Contracts Finder. GOV.UK. https://www.contractsfinder.service.gov.uk/notice/7c41c042-a30a-48ab-aad8-90cef615e1a1?origin=SearchResults&p=2

6. Register of Interests – Members of the House of Lords – Lord Deighton. UK Parliament. Retrieved May 16, 2024, from https://members.parliament.uk/members/lords/interests/register-of-lords-interests?SearchTerm=deighton&ShowAmendments=True

7. Provision Of Services To Support The UK Covid-19 Testing Strategy – Contracts Finder. (2020, December 14). Contracts Finder. GOV.UK. https://www.contractsfinder.service.gov.uk/notice/615ed22e-c062-4e57-af54-d7bd9f0c0aad?origin=SearchResults&p=1

8. The rollout of the Covid-19 vaccination programme in England. (2022, February 25). National Audit Office. https://www.nao.org.uk/wp-content/uploads/2022/02/The-rollout-of-the-Covid-19-vaccination-programme-in-England.pdf

9. Scott, R., & Williams, M. (2021, August 12). Secretive 'spy' Firm Met UK Minister To Discuss PPE Supply. OpenDemocracy. https://www.opendemocracy.net/en/opendemocracyuk/secretive-spy-firm-met-uk-minister-to-discuss-ppe-supply/

10. HAKLUYT & COMPANY LIMITED Filing History – Find And Update Company Information – GOV.UK. (n.d.). Companies House. GOV.UK. Retrieved May 16, 2024, from https://find-and-update.company-information.service.gov.uk/company/03481321/filing-history?page=2

11. Scott, R., & Williams, M. (2021, August 12). Secretive 'spy' Firm Met UK Minister To Discuss PPE Supply. OpenDemocracy. https://www.opendemocracy.net/en/opendemocracyuk/secretive-spy-firm-met-uk-minister-to-discuss-ppe-supply/

12. PPE Procurement In The Early Pandemic. (2021, November 17). GOV.UK. https://www.gov.uk/government/news/ppe-procurement-in-the-early-pandemic

13. BREAKING: Government Admits At Least four Ministers Used Private Emails For Government Business – Good Law Project. (2021, July 23). Good Law Project. https://goodlawproject.org/update/breaking-government-admits-trade-minister-greg-hands-and-ppe-tsar-lord-deighton-used-private-emails/

14. Supply Of Personal Protective Equipment For Healthcare Workers For The Care Of Patients With Suspected Or Confirmed Novel Coronavirus (Covid-19) – Contracts Finder. (2020b, December 2). Contracts Finder. GOV.UK. https://www.contractsfinder.service.gov.uk/notice/844bcb0e-124b-4586-ad32-6b7c302738e8?origin=SearchResults&p=1

15. Sequoia Capital China summary. Crunchbase. Retrieved May 16, 2024, from https://www.crunchbase.com/organization/sequoia-capital-china

16. Don Vieira Joins Hakluyt's Board Of Directors – Hakluyt. (2022, October). Hakluyt. https://hakluytandco.com/news/don-vieira-joins-hakluyts-board-of-directors/

17. Goodley, S. (2021, October 4). Tory Peer Did Not Declare Secret Offshore Investments, Leak Suggests. *The Guardian*. https://www.theguardian.com/news/2021/oct/04/tory-peer-did-not-declare-secret-offshore-investments-leak-suggests

18. Lord Markham CBE profile. (n.d.). GOV.UK. Retrieved May 16, 2024, from https://www.gov.uk/government/people/nick-markham

19. Baron Markham, Of East Horsley In The County Of Surrey. (2022, October 11). Peerage News. https://peeragenews.blogspot.com/2022/09/life-peerage-for-nicholas-markham.html

20. CIGNPOST DIAGNOSTICS LIMITED Overview – Find And Update Company Information – GOV.UK. (n.d.). Companies House. GOV.UK. Retrieved May 16, 2024, from https://find-and-update.company-information.service.gov.uk/company/12657158

21. 4-hour & Same-day PCR Tests Launched | Cignpost Diagnostics. (2022, February 3). Cignpost Diagnostics. https://www.cignpostdiagnostics.com/press-articles/expresstest-launches-new-4-hr-and-same-day-pcr-tests-for-international-travel

22. CIGNPOST DIAGNOSTICS LIMITED Overview – Find And Update Company Information – GOV.UK. (n.d.). Companies House. GOV.UK. Retrieved May 16, 2024, from https://find-and-update.company-information.service.gov.uk/company/12657158

23. pen Access UK: Monitor Lobbying Meetings With Government. (n.d.). Openaccess Transparency. Retrieved May 16, 2024, from https://openaccess.transparency.org.uk/?meeting=77964

24. 24Open Access UK: Monitor Lobbying Meetings With Government. (n.d.-b). Openaccess.Transparency.Org.UK. Retrieved May 16, 2024,

Notes

from https://openaccess.transparency.org.uk/?meeting=75948

25. Bryant, C. (2022, February 17). Chris Bryant: MPs Should Run A Mile From Groups Controlled By Lobbyists. OpenDemocracy. https://www.opendemocracy.net/en/dark-money-investigations/chris-bryant-all-party-parliamentary-groups-corporate-lobbyists/

26. Johnston, J. (2021, December 3). Covid Testing Company Sponsored Parliamentary Group Which Called For Additional Testing Requirements. Politics Home. https://www.politicshome.com/news/article/covid-testing-company-sponsored-parliamentary-group-which-called-for-additional-testing-requirements

27. Register of All-Party Parliamentary Groups. UK Parliament. Retrieved May 16, 2024, from https://www.parliament.uk/mps-lords-and-offices/standards-and-financial-interests/parliamentary-commissioner-for-standards/registers-of-interests/register-of-all-party-party-parliamentary-groups/

28. APPG On Business In A Pandemic (Covid) World Meetings. (n.d.). APPG Business Resilience. Retrieved May 16, 2024, from https://www.appgbusinessresilience.org/attendees

29. Business Resilience APPG (Defunct). (n.d.). Parallel Parliament. Retrieved May 16, 2024, from https://www.parallelparliament.co.uk/APPG/business-resilience

30. Office Of The Registrar Of Consultant Lobbyists – Client Profile. (n.d.). The Office of the Registrar of Consultant Lobbyists. Retrieved May 16, 2024, from https://orcl.my.site.com/CLR_Client_Profile?Id=a084J00000CeuXzQAJ

31. Mark MacGregor – Penta Formerly Hume Brophy. (n.d.). Penta Formerly Hume Brophy. Retrieved May 16, 2024, from https://humebrophy.com/people/mark-macgregor/

32. Mason, R. (23-1-23). Conservative Health Minister Has Big Stake In Covid Testing Firm. *The Guardian*. https://www.theguardian.com/politics/2023/jan/23/conservative-health-minister-stake-covid-nick-markham-cignpost-investments

33. PPE Expenditure – Question. (2023, January 25). TheyWorkForYou. https://www.theyworkforyou.com/lords/?id=2023-01-25b.210.0&s=CIGNPOST#g210.4

34. Sommerlad, N., & Scott, R. (2024, January 22). Tory Health Minister Hasn't Sold Stake In Covid Testing Firm A Year After Pledge. *The Mirror*. https://www.mirror.co.uk/news/politics/tory-health-minister-still-hasnt-31940908

35. Geoghegan, P., & Scott, R. (2021, January 20). Tory Donor Lord Ashcroft's Outsourcing Firm Lands £350m Vaccination

Contract. OpenDemocracy. https://www.opendemocracy.net/en/
dark-money-investigations/revealed-tory-donor-lord-ashcrofts-
outsourcing-firm-given-350m-vaccination-contract/

36. Managed Service Provision Of Workers To Support The National Testing
Programme. – Contracts Finder. (2021, January 19). Contracts Finder.
GOV.UK. https://www.contractsfinder.service.gov.uk/Notice/42762274-
14df-4ea6-8c82-a7484fe7b8c0

37. Lord Michael Ashcroft's political donations. The Electoral Commission.
Retrieved May 16, 2024, from http://bit.ly/45EMb0Q

38. IMPELLAM GROUP LIMITED Filing History – Find And Update
Company Information – GOV.UK. (n.d.). Companies House. GOV.
UK. Retrieved May 16, 2024, from https://find-and-update.company-
information.service.gov.uk/company/06511961/filing-history

39. MEDACS HEALTHCARE LIMITED Filing History – Find And
Update Company Information – GOV.UK. (n.d.). Companies House.
GOV.UK. Retrieved May 16, 2024, from https://find-and-update.
company-information.service.gov.uk/company/02518546/filing-history

40. Medacs Healthcare – Croydon Is Rated Inadequate By CQC – Care
Quality Commission. (2019, January 2). Care Quality Commission.
https://www.cqc.org.uk/news/releases/medacs-healthcare-croydon-rated-
inadequate-cqc

41. Peerages awarded to former UK prime ministers. (2023, November 21).
House of Lords Library. https://lordslibrary.parliament.uk/peerages-
awarded-to-former-prime-ministers/

42. Lex Greensill. (2024, May 17). Wikipedia. https://en.wikipedia.org/wiki/
Lex_Greensill

43. Markortoff, K. (2021, March 21). David Cameron Texted Rishi Sunak
To Get Covid Loans For Greensill, Says Report. *The Guardian*. https://
www.theguardian.com/politics/2021/mar/21/david-cameron-texted-rishi-
sunak-to-get-covid-loans-for-greensill-says-report

44. Neate, R. (2021, May 11). Greensill: The Scale Of David Cameron's
Lobbying Texts Revealed. *The Guardian*. https://www.theguardian.com/
business/2021/may/11/greensill-the-scale-of-david-camerons-lobbying-
texts-revealed

45. Neate, R. (2021, May 11). Greensill: The Scale Of David Cameron's
Lobbying Texts Revealed. *The Guardian*. https://www.theguardian.com/
business/2021/may/11/greensill-the-scale-of-david-camerons-lobbying-
texts-revealed

46. Allegretti, A. (2021, August 9). David Cameron Said To Have Made
About $10m From Greensill Capital. *The Guardian*. https://www.
theguardian.com/politics/2021/aug/09/david-cameron-said-made-about-

10m-greensill-capital-bbc

47. Kollewe, J. (2023, February 28). Credit Suisse 'seriously Breached' Obligations On Greensill, Says Regulator. *The Guardian.* https://www. theguardian.com/business/2023/feb/28/credit-suisse-greensill-swiss-bank-finma

48. Allegretti, A. (2021a, July 22). Why Was The Greensill Review Commissioned And What Did It Find? *The Guardian.* https://www. theguardian.com/business/2021/jul/22/why-was-the-greensill-review-commissioned-and-what-did-it-find

49. Lessons from Greensill Capital Sixth Report of Session 2021–22. (2021, July 14). House of Commons Treasury Committee. https://committees. parliament.uk/publications/6800/documents/72205/default/

50. Cowburn, A. (2021, August 11). Firm Won £123m Contract After David Cameron Urged Matt Hancock To Attend Genomics Conference. The Independent. https://www.independent.co.uk/news/uk/politics/david-cameron-contract-matt-hancock-b1900558.html

51. Davies, H., & Goodley, S. (2021, April 26). David Cameron Introduced Schoolfriend To Tory 'fixer' To Discuss Covid Tests. *The Guardian.* https:// www.theguardian.com/politics/2021/apr/26/david-cameron-introduced-schoolfriend-to-tory-fixer-to-discuss-covid-tests

Chapter 4: The brokers

1. INQ000144792 – Third Witness Statement Provided By Sir Christopher Stephen Wormald, On Behalf Of Department Of Health And Social Care, Dated 29/03/2023. UK Covid-19 Inquiry Archives. (2023, November 2). UK Covid-19 Inquiry. https://covid19.public-inquiry.uk/ documents/inq000144792-third-witness-statement-provided-by-sir-christopher-stephen-wormald-on-behalf-of-department-of-health-and-social-care-dated-29-03-2023/

2. Supply Of Personal Protective Equipment For Healthcare Workers For The Care Of Patients With Suspected Or Confirmed Novel Coronavirus (Covid-19) – Contracts Finder. (2021, March 29). Contracts Finder. GVO.UK. https://www.contractsfinder.service.gov.uk/Notice/22f31ba8-4c78-44d0-a6bc-42e299840b87

3. Patel, Mirza And The Middlemen – Good Law Project. (2021, May 28). Good Law Project. https://goodlawproject.org/update/patel-mirza-and-the-middlemen/

4. Supply Of Personal Protective Equipment For Healthcare Workers For The Care Of Patients With Suspected Or Confirmed Novel Coronavirus (Covid-19) – Contracts Finder. (2020, July 21). Contracts Finder. GOV. UK. https://www.contractsfinder.service.gov.uk/notice/8b9eb33b-7a55-

4112-8163-c6f3d1524910?origin=SearchResults&p=1

5. Kemp, P. (2021, April 20). Covid Contracts: PPE Fixer Who Was Tory Donor Named In Admin Error. BBC News. https://www.bbc.co.uk/news/uk-56667960

6. Samir Jassal LinkedIn profile. LinkedIn. Retrieved May 16, 2024, from https://www.linkedin.com/in/samir-jassal-32138b172/details/experience/

7. Wikipedia. (2024, May 17). East Ham (UK Parliament Constituency). Wikipedia. https://en.wikipedia.org/wiki/East_Ham_(UK_Parliament_constituency)

8. Election For The Constituency Of Feltham And Heston On 8 June 2017. (n.d.). UK Parliament. Retrieved May 16, 2024, from https://electionresults.parliament.uk/elections/875

9. £100m+ Contract For Ex-Number 10 Adviser – Good Law Project. (n.d.). Good Law Project. Retrieved May 16, 2024, from https://goodlawproject.org/case/100m-contract/

10. Letter before action under the pre-action protocol for judicial review dated 08 April 2020. (n.d.). Good Law Project. Retrieved May 16, 2024, from https://drive.google.com/file/d/1PlUvyzzpUIqpnuJGF8Un4npDn_nhaosm/view

11. Patel, Mirza And The Middlemen – Good Law Project. (2021, May 28). Good Law Project. https://goodlawproject.org/update/patel-mirza-and-the-middlemen/

12. 2021.04.22 –[redacted] – PAP Response And Disclosure.pdf. (n.d.). Good Law Project. Retrieved May 16, 2024, from https://drive.google.com/file/d/11nsbaxPuVLO0BHmCxzFA_cIxhgqB3NDJ/view

13. Supply Of Personal Protective Equipment For Healthcare Workers For The Care Of Patients With Suspected Or Confirmed Novel Coronavirus (Covid-19) – Contracts Finder. (2021, March 29). Contracts Finder. GVO.UK. https://www.contractsfinder.service.gov.uk/Notice/22f31ba8-4c78-44d0-a6bc-42e299840b

14. 2021.04.22 –[redacted] – PAP Response And Disclosure.pdf. (n.d.). Good Law Project. Retrieved May 16, 2024, from https://drive.google.com/file/d/11nsbaxPuVLO0BHmCxzFA_cIxhgqB3NDJ/view

15. Summary Of Investigation – ASJ Properties Limited – ORCL. (2022, September 26). The Office of the Registrar of Consultant Lobbyists. https://registrarofconsultantlobbyists.org.uk/summary-of-investigation-asj-properties-limited-asjp/

16. Samir Jassal donations to the Conservative Party. The Electoral Commission. Retrieved May 16, 2024, from http://bit.ly/473puFW

17. Councillor Details – Cllr Samir Jassal – Gravesham Borough Council. (n.d.). Gravesham Borough Council. Retrieved May 16, 2024, from

Notes

https://democracy.gravesham.gov.uk/mgUserInfo.aspx?UID=4369

18. Davies, R. (2022, April 1). Profits Jump For Patel-backed PPE Firm After It Won £216m Contracts. *The Guardian*. https://www.theguardian. com/business/2022/apr/01/profits-jump-for-patel-backed-ppe-direct-limited-after-it-won-216m-contracts#:~:text=Revenues%20at%20 Pharmaceuticals%20Direct%20Limited,this%20week%20at%20 Companies%20House.

19. Twitter thread by @JolyonMaugham (2021, June 25). Twitter.com. https://twitter.com/JolyonMaugham/status/1408490348184281099?s=20

20. Twitter post by @JolyonMaugham (2023, December 04). Twitter.com. https://twitter.com/JolyonMaugham/status/1731739242307473650?s=20

21. Wikipedia. (2024a, May 17). Black Cube. Wikipedia. https:// en.wikipedia.org/wiki/Black_Cube

22. Viner, K. (2021, July 23). The Pegasus Project: Why Investigations Like This Are At The Heart Of *The Guardian*'s Mission. *The Guardian*. https:// www.theguardian.com/news/2021/jul/23/pegasus-project-investigations-nso-spyware-mobile-phones

23. SUNBEAM CONSULTING LTD. Companies House. https://find-and-update.company-information.service.gov.uk/company/14017048/ persons-with-significant-control

24. Colbert, M. (2024, september 11). *Priti Patel took leadership donation from firm linked to PPE deal*. Good Law Project. fixerhttps://goodlawproject. org/priti-patel-took-leadership-donation-from-firm-linked-to-ppe-deal-fixer/

25. Scott, R. (2022, December 21). REVEALED: The Names Of Those Who Referred Covid Testing Firms Into The "VIP" Lane – Good Law Project. Good Law Project. https://goodlawproject.org/revealed-the-names-of-those-who-referred-covid-testing-firms-into-the-vip-lane/

26. UK Health Security Agency. Referrers to the Covid testing 'VIP' route. (n.d.). Good Law Project. Retrieved May 16, 2024, from https://drive. google.com/file/d/1i1DhMGaIvuQlfqn2tTUiBC0TcNy5rYll/view

27. Lawrence, F. (2023, May 18). Covid Contracts: Messages Reveal Extent Of Tory Donor Access To Matt Hancock. *The Guardian*. https://www. theguardian.com/politics/2023/may/18/covid-contracts-messages-reveal-extent-of-tory-donor-access-to-matt-hancock

28. Scott, R. (2023, May 18). EXCLUSIVE: WhatsApp Messages Reveal Matt Hancock Helped Tory Donor Win Covid Contract That Cost The Taxpayer £38m – Good Law Project. Good Law Project. https:// goodlawproject.org/exclusive-whatsapp-messages-reveal-matt-hancock-helped-tory-donor-win-covid-contract-that-cost-the-taxpayer-38m/

29. Settlement Agreement – Contracts Finder. (2021, June 4). Contracts

Finder. GOV.UK. https://www.contractsfinder.service.gov.uk/notice/0db50ff2-29d4-4ace-a48b-d008a1a1058e?origin=SearchResults&p=1

30. Lovett, S. (2021, April 29). Government 'wasted' £38.4m On Test And Trace Contract With Dubai-based Multinational. The Independent. https://www.independent.co.uk/news/health/test-and-trace-nhs-contract-uk-b1838329.html

31. Lawrence, F. (2023, May 18). Covid Contracts: Messages Reveal Extent Of Tory Donor Access To Matt Hancock. *The Guardian*. https://www.theguardian.com/politics/2023/may/18/covid-contracts-messages-reveal-extent-of-tory-donor-access-to-matt-hancock

32. Rapid Covid-19 Test, Oxsed RaViD Direct, Now In Use At Heathrow And Trials At Hong Kong International Airport | University Of Oxford. (2020, November 4). University of Oxford. https://www.ox.ac.uk/news/2020-11-04-rapid-covid-19-test-oxsed-ravid-direct-now-use-heathrow-and-trials-hong-kong

33. Mason, R. (2024, February 29). MP Calls For NCA To Consider Dealings Of Tory Donor Mohamed Amersi. *The Guardian*. https://www.theguardian.com/politics/2024/feb/29/mp-david-davis-calls-for-nca-to-consider-dealings-of-tory-donor-mohamed-amersi

34. Conn, D. (2021, May 18). Ministers 'lobbied' Officials Over PPE Contracts, Court Hears. *The Guardian*. https://www.theguardian.com/politics/2021/may/18/ministers-lobbied-officials-over-ppe-contracts-court-hears

35. 35.Smith, M. (2021, May 18). Bank Suspended Matt Hancock's PPE Deal Payments Fearing 'VIPs' Could Be Fraud. *The Mirror*. https://www.mirror.co.uk/news/politics/bank-suspended-matt-hancocks-ppe-24135963

36. Supply Of Personal Protective Equipment For Healthcare Workers For The Care Of Patients With Suspected Or Confirmed Novel Coronavirus (Covid-19) – Contracts Finder. (2020b, July 27). Contracts Finder. GOV.UK. https://www.contractsfinder.service.gov.uk/notice/411d0ae0-29e0-4f26-b4b9-a9dfcd8bb974?origin=SearchResults&p=1

37. Twitter thread b7 @jolyonmaugham. (2020, August 6). Twitter.com. https://twitter.com/JolyonMaugham/status/1291244610539462656?s=20

38. 2020.07.29 –[redacted] – Letter Of Response By GLD.pdf. (1970, January 1). Good Law Project. https://drive.google.com/file/d/1oyYEIwe1-N-XH_IWqX5B8osOSJBYchTQ/view

39. PPE Procurement In The Early Pandemic. (2021, November 17). GOV.UK. https://www.gov.uk/government/news/ppe-procurement-in-the-early-pandemic

Notes

40. PROSPERMILL Filing History – Find And Update Company Information – GOV.UK. (n.d.). Companies House. GOV.UK. Retrieved May 17, 2024, from https://find-and-update.company-information. service.gov.uk/company/11807105/filing-history

41. Kirk, T. (2021, May 18). Hedge Fund 'fast-tracked To £252m PPE Deal Despite Red Flags.' Evening Standard. https://www.standard.co.uk/news/ uk/ayanda-ppe-high-court-pestfix-good-law-project-b935795.html

42. Kirk, T. (2021, May 18). Hedge Fund 'fast-tracked To £252m PPE Deal Despite Red Flags.' Evening Standard. https://www.standard.co.uk/news/ uk/ayanda-ppe-high-court-pestfix-good-law-project-b935795.html

43. 2020.07.29 –[redacted] – Letter Of Response By GLD.pdf. (1970, January 1). Good Law Project. https://drive.google.com/file/ d/1oyYEIwe1-N-XH_lWqX5B8osOSJBYchTQ/view

44. Twitter post by @GoodLawProject. (2021, May 19). Twitter.com. https:// twitter.com/GoodLawProject/status/1395062212507717632?s=20

45. Twitter post by @GoodLawProject. (2021, May 19). Twitter.com.https:// twitter.com/GoodLawProject/status/1394973409017221122?s=20

46. Smith, M. (2021, May 18). Bank Suspended Matt Hancock's PPE Deal Payments Fearing 'VIPs' Could Be Fraud. *The Mirror*. https://www.mirror. co.uk/news/politics/bank-suspended-matt-hancocks-ppe-24135963

47. 2020.07.29 –[redacted] – Letter Of Response By GLD.pdf. (1970, January 1). Good Law Project. https://drive.google.com/file/ d/1oyYEIwe1-N-XH_lWqX5B8osOSJBYchTQ/view

48. Brooks, R. (n.d.). Profit of Doom. Private Eye. Retrieved May 17, 2024, from https://www.private-eye.co.uk/pictures/special_reports/profits-of-doom.pdf

49. 49Supply Of Personal Protective Equipment For Healthcare Workers For The Care Of Patients With Suspected Or Confirmed Novel Coronavirus (Covid-19) – Contracts Finder. (2020a, June 23). Contracts Finder. GOV. UK. https://www.contractsfinder.service.gov.uk/notice/2059f09e-5b4f-49d4-afa8-2d54f0adf51b?origin=SearchResults&p=1

50. Home – Euthenia Investments. (n.d.). Euthenia Investments. Retrieved May 17, 2024, from https://eutheniainvestments.co.uk/

51. EUTHENIA INVESTMENTS LTD Filing History – Find And Update Company Information – GOV.UK. (n.d.). Companies House. GOV.UK. Retrieved May 17, 2024, from https://find-and-update. company-information.service.gov.uk/company/12311110/filing-history?page=2

52. PPE Procurement In The Early Pandemic. (2021b, November 17). GOV.UK. https://www.gov.uk/government/news/ppe-procurement-in-the-early-pandemic#:~:text=Those%20to%20whom%20contracts%20

were,was%20processed%20through%20the%20mailbox.

53. MP's Daughter Threatened To Sue For 'VIP Lane' Commission –
Good Law Project. (2023, February 27). Good Law Project. https://
goodlawproject.org/mps-daughter-threatened-to-sue-for-vip-lane-
commission/

Chapter 5: Private health firms and the former PM

1. NHS England » NHS Strikes Major Deal To Expand Hospital Capacity
To Battle Coronavirus. (2020, March 21). NHS England. https://www.
england.nhs.uk/2020/03/nhs-strikes-major-deal-to-expand-hospital-
capacity-to-battle-coronavirus/

2. 492193-2020 – Result. (n.d.). TED. Retrieved May 17, 2024, from
https://ted.europa.eu/en/notice/-/detail/492193-2020

3. Letter to Regional Directors/Regional Leadership Teams. subject:
Covid-19: Partnership working with the Independent Sector Providers
and the Independent Healthcare Providers Network (IHPN). dated 24
March 2020. (n.d.). NHS England. Retrieved May 17, 2024, from https://
www.ihpn.org.uk/wp-content/uploads/2020/03/IHPN-Partnership-
Letter-to-system-24-March-2020.pdf

4. Davies, R. (2021, May 5). Ministers Urged To Reveal Details Of £2bn
Covid Deals With Private Health Firms. *The Guardian*. https://www.
theguardian.com/politics/2021/may/05/uk-government-publish-details-
covid-contracts-private-healthcare-firms

5. Scott, R. (2021, November 3). EXCLUSIVE: Private Hospitals Were
Paid Over £1.5 Billion During The Pandemic – Good Law Project.
Good Law Project. https://goodlawproject.org/private-hospitals-billion-
pandemic/

6. 'Williams, M., Corderoy, J., Geoghegan, P., & Taylor, J. (2021, July 6). 'No
Record' Of Matt Hancock Meeting Tory Donor Who Owns Stake In
£346m Covid Contract. OpenDemocracy. https://www.opendemocracy.
net/en/dark-money-investigations/no-record-of-matt-hancock-meeting-
tory-donor-who-owns-stake-in-346m-covid-contract/

7. Davies, R. (2021, May 5). Ministers Urged To Reveal Details Of £2bn
Covid Deals With Private Health Firms. *The Guardian*. https://www.
theguardian.com/politics/2021/may/05/uk-government-publish-details-
covid-contracts-private-healthcare-firms

8. Ryan, S., Rowland, D., McCoy, D., & Leys, C. (2021, November). For
Whose Benefit? NHS England's contract with the private hospital
sector in the first year of the pandemic. Centre for Health and the Public
Interest. https://chpi-fd3a752d575a6d9748da-endpoint.azureedge.net/
wp-content/uploads/2021/09/CHPI-For-Whose-Benefit_.pdf

Notes

9. ICO Decision notice. Reference: IC-113081-Z9M4. (2021, October 20). Information Commissioner's Office. https://ico.org.uk/media/action-weve-taken/decision-notices/2021/4018849/ic-113081-z9m4.pdf

10. Scott, R. (2021, November 3). EXCLUSIVE: Private Hospitals Were Paid Over £1.5 Billion During The Pandemic – Good Law Project. Good Law Project. https://goodlawproject.org/private-hospitals-billion-pandemic/

11. NHS Increasing Capacity Framework – Contracts Finder. (2021, February 4). Contracts Finder. GOV.UK. https://www.contractsfinder.service.gov.uk/notice/4396060d-ae84-4cb2-af0a-54e74fa5f24a?origin=SearchResults&p=1

12. NHS England » Payments Over £25k Reports: 2022. (2023, September 22). NHS England. https://www.england.nhs.uk/publication/payments-over-25k-reports-2022/

13. Lord Nash, Registered Interests. UK Parliament. Retrieved May 17, 2024, from https://members.parliament.uk/member/4270/registeredinterests

14. Dunn, W. (2024, February 23). Revealed: The Tory Peer Linked To £3.8bn In Government Contracts. New Statesman. https://www.newstatesman.com/politics/2024/02/revealed-tory-peer-linked-billion-government-contracts

15. The Phoenix Partnership (Leeds) Ltd donations to political parties. The Electoral Commission. Retrieved May 17, 2024, from http://bit.ly/3VcSPXe

16. Government Gives Tory Donor £137m In Hidden Payments – Good Law Project. (2023, September 20). Good Law Project. https://goodlawproject.org/government-gives-tory-donor-137m-in-hidden-payments/

17. About Us. (n.d.). TPP. Retrieved May 17, 2024, from https://tpp-uk.com/about-us/

18. GPITF Framework Point Of Care Supplier Extension 2022-23 – Contracts Finder. (2024, February 13). Contracts Finder. GOV.UK. https://www.contractsfinder.service.gov.uk/notice/a08d1e88-6976-4a8c-9f49-d3f2420b2d29?origin=SearchResults&p=1

19. Twitter post from @TPP_SystmOne. (2022, December 13). Twitter.com. https://x.com/TPP_SystmOne/status/1602615963572211712

20. THE PHOENIX PARTNERSHIP (LEEDS) LTD Filing History – Find And Update Company Information – GOV.UK. (n.d.). Companies House. GOV.UK. Retrieved May 17, 2024, from https://find-and-update.company-information.service.gov.uk/company/04077829/filing-history

21. Open Access UK: Monitor Lobbying Meetings With Government. (n.d.). Https://Openaccess.Transparency.Org.Uk/. Retrieved May 17, 2024, from

https://openaccess.transparency.org.uk/?meeting=84817

22. Mason, R., Weaver, M., & Dyer, H. (2024, March 11). Biggest Tory Donor Said Looking At Diane Abbott Makes You 'want To Hate All Black Women.' *The Guardian*. https://www.theguardian.com/politics/2024/mar/11/biggest-tory-donor-looking-diane-abbott-hate-all-black-women

23. The Phoenix Partnership (Leeds) Ltd donations to political parties. The Electoral Commission. Retrieved May 17, 2024, from http://bit.ly/3UB1BOC

24. View Donation – The Electoral Commission. (2023, September 6). The Electoral Commission. https://search.electoralcommission.org.uk/English/Donations/C0570256

25. Mason, R., Weaver, M., & Dyer, H. (2024, March 11). Biggest Tory Donor Said Looking At Diane Abbott Makes You 'want To Hate All Black Women.' *The Guardian*. https://www.theguardian.com/politics/2024/mar/11/biggest-tory-donor-looking-diane-abbott-hate-all-black-women

26. Mason, R., Weaver, M., & Dyer, H. (2024, March 11). Biggest Tory Donor Said Looking At Diane Abbott Makes You 'want To Hate All Black Women.' *The Guardian*. https://www.theguardian.com/politics/2024/mar/11/biggest-tory-donor-looking-diane-abbott-hate-all-black-women

27. Mason, R., Weaver, M., & Dyer, H. (2024, March 11). Biggest Tory Donor Said Looking At Diane Abbott Makes You 'want To Hate All Black Women.' *The Guardian*. https://www.theguardian.com/politics/2024/mar/11/biggest-tory-donor-looking-diane-abbott-hate-all-black-women

28. Neilan, C. (2024, March 14). Exclusive: Tory Party "sitting On" Further £5m From Disgraced Donor Frank Hester. Tortoise. https://www.tortoisemedia.com/2024/03/14/exclusive-tory-party-accepts-a-further-5m-from-controversial-frank-hester/

29. Weaver, M., & Campbell, D. (2024, March 19). NHS England Chief Condemns Frank Hester's 'racist, Sexist And Violent' Remarks. *The Guardian*. https://www.theguardian.com/business/2024/mar/19/nhs-england-chief-condemns-frank-hester-racist-sexist-and-violent-remarks

30. Scott, R. (2024, April 23). Firm Owned By Tory Donor Frank Hester Lands Another £4.4m NHS Contract. Torchlight: Russell Scott's Substack. https://russellscott.substack.com/p/firm-owned-by-tory-donor-frank-hester

31. Twitter post by @HesterObe. (2023, November 14). Twitter. https://x.com/HesterObe/status/1724389788248133770

Notes

32. Twitter post by @RussellScott1. (2024, March 25). Twitter.https://x.com/ RussellScott1/status/1772241757314417108

33. Adu, A. (2023, May 19). Rishi Sunak's Family Fortune Falls By £200m In Sunday Times Rich List. *The Guardian*. https://www.theguardian.com/ politics/2023/may/19/rishi-sunak-akshata-murty-family-fortune-falls-by-200m-in-rich-list#:~:text=Sunak%2C%20a%20former%20hedge%20 fund,from%20%C2%A3730m%20in%202022.

34. Riley, H. (2024, February 12). Rishi Sunak's Wife's Firm Infosys Received 50% Boost In Public Sector Invoices In 2023. LBC. https://www.lbc. co.uk/news/akshata-murty-infosys-contracts/

35. Contract Finder. GOV.UK. Retrieved May 17, 2024, from https://www. contractsfinder.service.gov.uk/Search/Results

36. Geoghegan, P. (2024, January 28). Revealed: Sunak Wife's Family Firm In Line For Millions In New Public Contracts. Democracy for Sale. https:// democracyforsale.substack.com/p/sunak-family-firm-infosys-public-contracts)

37. Scott, R. (2023, November 8). Infosys – The Company Founded By PM's Father-in-law Lands New Public Sector Contracts. Torchlight: Russell Scott's Substack. https://russellscott.substack.com/p/infosys-the-company-founded-by-pms

38. INTELLIGENT AUTOMATION (SBS10137) – Contracts Finder. (2023, December 16). Contracts Finder. GOV.UK. https://www. contractsfinder.service.gov.uk/notice/e2dd4146-a289-4d44-8482-4787fb69831e?origin=SearchResults&p=1

39. Hunt, S. (2023, October 12). Rishi Sunak's Wife Earns More Than All Labour MPs Combined After £6.8m Dividend. Evening Standard. https://www.standard.co.uk/business/rishi-sunak-s-wife-earns-more-than-all-labour-mps-combined-after-fresh-dividend-b1113119.html

40. Helm, T., & Dhillon, A. (2023, August 26). Rishi Sunak Faces Fresh Conflict Of Interest Row Over India Trade Talks. *The Guardian*. https:// www.theguardian.com/politics/2023/aug/26/rishi-sunak-faces-fresh-conflict-of-interest-row-over-india-trade-talks

41. Walker, J. (2023, August 2). Rishi Sunak's family firm Infosys signed $1.5B deal with BP. The National. https://www.thenational.scot/ news/23697572.rishi-sunaks-family-firm-infosys-signed-1-5b-deal-bp/

42. Scott, R. (2023, November 8). Infosys – The Company Founded By PM's Father-in-law Lands New Public Sector Contracts. Torchlight: Russell Scott's Substack. https://russellscott.substack.com/p/infosys-the-company-founded-by-pms

43. Sommerlad, N., & Scott, R. (2023, December 9). Fund Set Up By Top Tories Is Huge Investor In Firm Behind Sunak Family Fortune.

The Mirror. https://www.mirror.co.uk/news/politics/fund-set-up-top-tories-31637769

44. Sommerlad, N., Scott, R., & Geoghegan, P. (2024, February 3). Top Tory Accused Of Offering 'VIP Lane' For Rishi Sunak's Wife's Firm In UK. *The Mirror*. https://www.mirror.co.uk/news/politics/top-tory-accused-offering-vip-32040731

45. List of Minister' interest. (2023, December). INDEPENDENT ADVISER ON MINISTERS' INTERESTS. https://assets.publishing.service.gov.uk/media/657add84095987000d95e0ca/List_of_Ministers__Interests_-_December_2023.pdf

46. Prime Minister's Schedule Of Taxable Sources Of Income And Gains. (2023, March 22). GOV.UK. https://www.gov.uk/government/collections/prime-ministers-schedule-of-taxable-sources-of-income-and-gains

47. Prime Minister's Schedule Of Taxable Sources Of Income And Gains. (2023, March 22). GOV.UK. https://www.gov.uk/government/collections/prime-ministers-schedule-of-taxable-sources-of-income-and-gains

48. Barr, B. (2022, November 8). Register Of Members' Financial Interests | Institute For Government. Institute For Government. https://www.instituteforgovernment.org.uk/explainer/register-members-financial-interests

49. Dyer, H. (2023, December 14). Do Blind Trusts For UK Ministers Really Prevent Conflicts Of Interest? *The Guardian*. https://www.theguardian.com/money/2023/dec/14/are-blind-trusts-more-than-uk-tool-that-gives-perception-of-probity

50. Scott, R. (2023, February 6). Sunak-linked Hedge Fund Sees Pandemic Profits Soar To £109m – Good Law Project. Good Law Project. https://goodlawproject.org/sunak-linked-hedge-fund-sees-pandemic-profits-soar-to-109m/

51. Theleme Partners Portfolio | Patrick Degorce 13F Holdings & Trades. (n.d.). HedgeFollow. Retrieved May 17, 2024, from https://hedgefollow.com/funds/Theleme+Partners

52. UK Cements 10-year-partnership With Moderna In Major Boost For Vaccines And Research. (2022, December 22). GOV.UK. https://www.gov.uk/government/news/uk-cements-10-year-partnership-with-moderna-in-major-boost-for-vaccines-and-research

53. A Review Of The Vaccine Taskforce. (2023, August 29). GOV.UK. https://www.gov.uk/government/publications/a-review-of-the-vaccine-taskforce/a-review-of-the-vaccine-taskforce#key-facts-and-figures

54. Garside, J. (2020, November 17). Rishi Sunak Refuses To Say If He Will Profit From Moderna Covid Vaccine. *The Guardian*. https://www.theguardian.com/politics/2020/nov/17/rishi-sunak-refuses-to-say-if-he-will-profit-from-moderna-covid-vaccine

55. Scott, R. (2024, December 3). Rishi Sunak Accused of Having 'Something to Hide' After Burying Post-Downing Street Interests Behind Financial 'Firewall'. *Byline Times.* https://bylinetimes.com/2024/12/03/rishi-sunak-accused-of-having-something-to-hide-after-burying-post-downing-street-interests-behind-financial-firewall/

Chapter 6: Up in smoke

1. The Government Did Not Spend £37 Billion On The NHS Test And Trace App – Full Fact. (2023, April 6). Full Fact. https://fullfact.org/health/NHS-test-and-trace-app-37-billion-instagram/
2. NQ000144792 – Third Witness Statement Provided By Sir Christopher Stephen Wormald, On Behalf Of Department Of Health And Social Care, Dated 29/03/2023. UK Covid-19 Inquiry Archives. (2023, November 2). UK Covid-19 Inquiry. https://covid19.public-inquiry.uk/documents/inq000144792-third-witness-statement-provided-by-sir-christopher-stephen-wormald-on-behalf-of-department-of-health-and-social-care-dated-29-03-2023/
3. Supply Of Personal Protective Equipment For Healthcare Workers For The Care Of Patients With Suspected Or Confirmed Novel Coronavirus (Covid-19) – Contracts Finder. (2021, March 29). Contracts Finder. GOV.UK. https://www.contractsfinder.service.gov.uk/Notice/22f31ba8-4c78-44d0-a6bc-42e299840b87
4. Supply Of FFP3 Respirators – Contracts Finder. (2020, November 25). Contracts Finder. GOV.UK. https://www.contractsfinder.service.gov.uk/notice/8a31d06e-1dc6-4b62-ba99-1deb33a77c6b?origin=SearchResults&p=1
5. Investigation into the management of PPE contracts. (2022, March 30). National Audit Office. https://www.nao.org.uk/wp-content/uploads/2022/03/Investigation-into-the-management-of-PPE-contracts.pdf
6. Scott, R. (2022, February 1). PPE To Go Up In Smoke – Literally – As The Bill For Waste Tops £10 Billion – Good Law Project. Good Law Project. https://goodlawproject.org/ppe-to-go-up-in-smoke/
7. DHSC Annual Report And Accounts: 2020 To 2021. (2022, January 31). GOV.UK. https://www.gov.uk/government/publications/dhsc-annual-report-and-accounts-2020-to-2021
8. Nunis, V. (2020, November 14). Felixstowe Port In 'chaos' As Christmas And Brexit Loom. BBC News. https://www.bbc.co.uk/news/business-54908129
9. Sommerlad, N., Smith, L., & Scott, R. (2021, November 5). Piles Of Unused PPE Cost £1m A Day To Store In 'grotesque Waste Of Public

Money.' *The Mirror*. https://www.mirror.co.uk/news/politics/piles-unused-ppe-costing-1million-25391211

10. Stephens, M. (2020, December 18). Thousands of shipping containers of surplus PPE moved to railway station after blocking up ports. *The Telegraph* https://www.telegraph.co.uk/news/2020/12/18/thousands-shipping-containers-surplus-ppe-moved-railway-station/

11. DHSC spending over £25,000. (n.d.). GOV.UK. Retrieved May 17, 2024, from https://www.google.com/url?q=https://www.gov.uk/government/collections/spending-over-25-000--2&sa=D&source=docs&ust=1715961351481197&usg=AOvVaw3jdACbW40xWpp5JL79cJ_y

12. PPE Procurement In The Early Pandemic. (2021, November 17). GOV.UK. https://www.gov.uk/government/news/ppe-procurement-in-the-early-pandemic

13. Half Of VIP Lane Companies Supplied PPE Worth £1 Billion That Was Not Fit For Purpose – Spotlight On Corruption. (2022, February 11). Spotlight On Corruption. https://www.spotlightcorruption.org/half-of-vip-lane-companies-supplied-ppe-worth-1-billion-that-was-not-fit-for-purpose/

14. Uniserve – Contracts Finder. (2021, April 21). Contracts Finder. GOV.UK. https://www.contractsfinder.service.gov.uk/notice/b43b1b5d-adac-45ad-9753-5d30b14d8335?origin=SearchResults&p=1

15. UNISERVE LIMITED Filing History – Find And Update Company Information – GOV.UK. (n.d.). Companies House. GOV.UK. Retrieved May 17, 2024, from https://find-and-update.company-information.service.gov.uk/company/01826635/filing-history

16. PPE Expenditure – Question. (2023, January 25). TheyWorkForYou. https://www.theyworkforyou.com/lords/?id=2023-01-25b.210.0&s=%22markham%22+%22ppe%22#g210.2

17. committees.parliament.uk/publications/42056/documents/209249/default/ Wormald, C. (2023, November 7). Letter to Dame Meg Hiller MP, Chair of Public Accounts Committee. Department of Health and Social Care. https://committees.parliament.uk/publications/42056/documents/209249/default/

18. RM6282 Clipper Award – PPE Disposal – Contracts Finder. (2022, December 6). Contracts Finder. GOV.UK. https://www.contractsfinder.service.gov.uk/Notice/f3b76c36-90f1-4c30-8c72-beaaffec6ee5

19. Scott, R. (2022b, December 12). REVEALED: Tory Donor's Company Awarded £4.5 Million Government Contract To Take Care Of Mountain Of Unusable PPE Waste – Good Law Project. Good Law Project. https://goodlawproject.org/revealed-tory-donors-company-awarded-4-5-million-government-contract-to-take-care-of-mountain-of-unusable-ppe-waste/

20. Smith, B. (2022, April 8). EXCL: DHSC To Pay Up To £35m To Dispose Of Unused Pandemic PPE. Civil Service World. https://www.civilserviceworld.com/professions/article/excl-dhsc-to-pay-up-to-35m-to-dispose-of-burn-recycle-unused-pandemic-ppe-covid

21. Siddle, J., & White, C. (2023, January 16). EXCLUSIVE: Tory donor's firm paid £11m to deliver PPE now gets £4.5m of taxpayer money to DESTROY it. The Mirror. https://www.mirror.co.uk/news/politics/tory-donors-firm-paid-11m-28956268

22. Watt, H. (2015, May 4). Redirecting. The Guardian. https://www.google.com/url?q=https://www.theguardian.com/politics/2015/may/04/tories-leaders-group-donor-club-david-cameron-conservatives-dinners&sa=D&source=docs&ust=1715963211717496&usg=AOvVaw35nBnDcQ6mEi7yAU8bD-Ml

23. Smith, M. (2024, March 1). Inside The Tory Winter Ball Where Rich Donors Paid £25k To Dine With Jeremy Hunt. The Mirror. https://www.mirror.co.uk/news/politics/inside-tory-winter-ball-wealthy-32250143

24. Smith, B. (2022, April 8). EXCL: DHSC To Pay Up To £35m To Dispose Of Unused Pandemic PPE. Civil Service World. https://www.civilserviceworld.com/professions/article/excl-dhsc-to-pay-up-to-35m-to-dispose-of-burn-recycle-unused-pandemic-ppe-covid

25. Contracts Finder. (2024, March 25). Contracts Finder. GOV.UK. https://www.contractsfinder.service.gov.uk/notice/2b9fa945-a9a1-4112-84c8-eeba3a1bd689?origin=SearchResults&p=1

26. Thomas, J. (2023, November 08). Stories. Logical next step. TheOwnerBreeder.com. https://theownerbreeder.com/stories/logical-next-step/

27. Half Of VIP Lane Companies Supplied PPE Worth £1 Billion That Was Not Fit For Purpose – Spotlight On Corruption. (2022, February 11). Spotlight On Corruption. https://www.spotlightcorruption.org/half-of-vip-lane-companies-supplied-ppe-worth-1-billion-that-was-not-fit-for-purpose/

28. 28 Coronavirus: Protective Clothing, Question for Department of Health and Social Care, UIN HL2327, tabled on 18 August 2021. UK Parliament. Retrieved May 17, 2024, from https://questions-statements.parliament.uk/written-questions/detail/2021-08-18/hl2327

29. Grafton-Green, P. (2021, April 21). Govt PPE And Covid Contracts Worth 3.7bn Raise Corruption Concerns, Report Says. LBC. https://www.lbc.co.uk/news/govt-ppe-and-covid-contracts-worth-37bn-raise-corruption-concerns-report-says/

30. PM Call With UK's Leading Manufacturers: 16 March 2020. (2020, March 16). GOV.UK. https://www.gov.uk/government/news/pm-call-with-uks-leading-manufacturers-16-march-2020

31. Rt Hon Boris Johnson MP Meetings, January To March 2020 – GOV. UK. (2020, July 30). Cabinet Office. https://assets.publishing.service.gov. uk/media/5f21984de90e071a5b04b4d8/Rt-Hon-Boris-Johnson-MP-meetings-January-to-March-2020.csv/preview

32. Investigation into how government increased the number of ventilators available to the NHS in response to Covid-19. (2020, September 30). National Audit Office. https://www.nao.org.uk/wp-content/uploads/2020/09/Investigation-into-how-the-Government-increased-the-number-of-ventilators.pdf

33. James Dyson Foundation donations to political parties. The Electoral Commission. Retrieved May 17, 2024, from http://bit.ly/3UEKSKk

34. Bamford donations to political parties. The Electoral Commission. Retrieved May 17, 2024, from http://bit.ly/45DGAt3

35. Sommerlad, N. (2023, January 10). Boris Johnson Living In Donor's £20m Home On One Of UK's Most Expensive Streets. *The Mirror.* https://www.mirror.co.uk/news/politics/shameless-boris-johnson-living-20m-28922635?_ga=2.151811386.2093599896.1710805456-762803238.1590447098#source=breaking-news

36. Boris Johnson, Former MP, Uxbridge And South Ruislip. (n.d.). TheyWorkForYou. Retrieved May 17, 2024, from www.theyworkforyou.com/mp/10999/boris_johnson/uxbridge_and_south_ruislip#register

37. INQ000048399_0001-0003 – Extract of Dominic Cummings' WhatsApp messages from 'CSA-CMO-Matt-PM-Dom', dated 07/11/2020. – UK Covid-19 Inquiry (covid19.public-inquiry.uk)

38. INQ000048399_0001-0003 – Extract Of Dominic Cummings' WhatsApp Messages From 'CSA-CMO-Matt-PM-Dom', Dated 07/11/2020. UK Covid-19 Inquiry Archives. (2024, February 16). UK Covid-19 Inquiry. https://covid19.public-inquiry.uk/documents/inq000048399_0001-0003-extract-of-dominic-cummings-whatsapp-messages-from-csa-cmo-matt-pm-dom-dated-07-11-2020/

39. Rapid Manufacture Ventilator System-Design Agreement For The Covent Model – Contracts Finder. (2023, February 28). Contracts Finder. GOV.UK. https://www.contractsfinder.service.gov.uk/notice/1eae0061-daf4-496c-8a19-7fd2c9d69a2b?origin=SearchResults&p=1

40. JCB JOINS NATIONAL CALL TO ACTION OVER VENTILATOR SHORTAGE. (2020, March 30). JCB.Com. https://www.jcb.com/en-gb/news/2020/03/jcb-joins-national-call-to-action-over-ventilator-shortage

41. Jack, S. (2020, March 25). Coronavirus: Government Orders 10,000 Ventilators From Dyson. BBC News. https://www.bbc.co.uk/news/business-52043767

42. INQ000106519 – Cabinet Office Website Publication Titled 'Ventilator Challenge Hailed A Success As UK Production Finishes', Dated 04/07/2020 UK Covid-19 Inquiry Archives. (2024, February 16). UK Covid-19 Inquiry. https://covid19.public-inquiry.uk/documents/inq000106519-cabinet-office-website-publication-titled-ventilator-challenge-hailed-a-success-as-uk-production-finishes-dated-04-07-2020/

43. Dawkins, D. (2020, April 24). Billionaire James Dyson Told Thanks But No Thanks–Ventilator Order Spiked By Government Following Reports Of PR 'Point Scoring'. Forbes. https://www.forbes.com/sites/daviddawkins/2020/04/24/billionaire-james-dyson-told-thanks-but-no-thanksventilator-order-spiked-by-government-following-reports-of-pr-point-scoring/

44. Cabinet Office: Spend Data Over £25,000. (2013, July 4). GOV.UK. https://www.gov.uk/government/publications/cabinet-office-spend-data

45. Provision Of Rapid Manufacture Ventilator Systems (RMVS) Resale And Disposal Of Surplus Components – Contracts Finder. (2023, February 24). Contracts Finder. GOV.UK. https://www.contractsfinder.service.gov.uk/notice/3750a747-e8f1-4f33-bdab-e33255ec0070?origin=SearchResults&p=2

46. Boris Johnson Told Sir James Dyson By Text He Would 'fix' Tax Issue. (2021, April 21). BBC News. https://www.bbc.co.uk/news/uk-politics-56819137

47. Ward, E. (2021, April 21). 'Sleeze, Sleeze, Sleeze' – Keir Starmer Accuses Government Of Cronyism. LBC. https://www.lbc.co.uk/news/starmer-and-johnson-clash-over-pms-pledge-to-fix-tax-for-dyson-workers-in-pandem/

48. Hardinges, N. (2021, April 22). 'Holy Trinity' Of Ventilator Callers Leave James O'Brien 'appalled At Government Cronyism'. LBC. https://www.lbc.co.uk/radio/presenters/james-obrien/three-ventilator-callers-james-obrien-appalled-government-cronyism-nhs-dyson/

49. Scott, R. (2025, March 05). Michael Gove Told Officials to Buy 10,000 Ventilators From Dyson During Pandemic in 'Affront' to Procurement Rules, Byline Times. https://bylinetimes.com/2025/03/05/michael-gove-told-officials-to-buy-10000-ventilators-from-dyson-during-pandemic-in-affront-to-procurement-rules/

50. Scott, R. (2023, February 9). WE WON: Government Commits To Publishing £248m Missing Covid Contracts After Breaching Transparency Guidelines – Good Law Project. Good Law Project. https://goodlawproject.org/we-won-government-commits-to-publishing-248m-missing-covid-contracts-after-breaching-transparency-guidelines

51. Investigation into how government increased the number of ventilators

available to the NHS in response to Covid-19. (2020, September 30). National Audit Office. https://www.nao.org.uk/wp-content/uploads/2020/09/Investigation-into-how-the-Government-increased-the-number-of-ventilators.pdf

52. Campbell, D. (2020, September 30). Covid: UK Spent £569m On 20,900 Ventilators But Most Remain Unused. *The Guardian*. https://www.theguardian.com/world/2020/sep/30/uk-spent-569m-on-20900-ventilators-for-covid-care-but-most-remain-unused

53. DHSC: P&P – MedTech – Auction Requirement (Income) – Contracts Finder. (2023, December 22). Contracts Finder. GOV.UK. https://www.contractsfinder.service.gov.uk/notice/ad43fff2-7216-4b7f-9885-59edce4e6fc3?origin=SearchResults&p=1

54. Sommerlad, N., & Scott, R. (2024, January 28). Thousands Of Covid Ventilators Bought For £50k Flogged Off For As Little As £100. *The Mirror*. https://www.mirror.co.uk/news/uk-news/thousands-covid-ventilators-bought-50k-31988459

55. Purchase Of Mechanical Ventilators – Contracts Finder. (2021, March 8). Contracts Finder. https://www.contractsfinder.service.gov.uk/notice/fecd5282-bcbc-4bc4-87b2-09b42ba64f43?origin=SearchResults&p=1

56. Investigation into how government increased the number of ventilators available to the NHS in response to Covid-19. (2020, September 30). National Audit Office. https://www.nao.org.uk/wp-content/uploads/2020/09/Investigation-into-how-the-Government-increased-the-number-of-ventilators.pdf

57. Supply Of Personal Protective Equipment For Healthcare Workers For The Care Of Patients With Suspected Or Confirmed Novel Coronavirus (Covid-19) – Contracts Finder. (2020, December 2). Contracts Finder. GOV.UK. https://www.contractsfinder.service.gov.uk/notice/51bf1d3a-89a9-42d2-bd81-5b24e92ee278?origin=SearchResults&p=1

58. PPE Procurement In The Early Pandemic. (2021, November 17). GOV.UK. https://www.gov.uk/government/news/ppe-procurement-in-the-early-pandemic

59. Half Of VIP Lane Companies Supplied PPE Worth £1 Billion That Was Not Fit For Purpose – Spotlight On Corruption. (2022, February 11). Spotlight On Corruption. https://www.spotlightcorruption.org/half-of-vip-lane-companies-supplied-ppe-worth-1-billion-that-was-not-fit-for-purpose/

60. Turning Tory Waste Into Shards Of Hope – Good Law Project. (2024, February 14). Good Law Project. https://goodlawproject.org/turning-tory-waste-into-shards-of-hope/

61. DHSC Annual Report And Accounts: 2021 To 2022. (2023, January 26).

GOV.UK. https://www.gov.uk/government/publications/dhsc-annual-report-and-accounts-2021-to-2022

62. Hall, R., & Campbell, D. (2023, January 26). Department Of Health Wasted £15bn On Unused Covid Supplies, Watchdog Finds. *The Guardian*. https://www.theguardian.com/society/2023/jan/26/department-of-health-wasted-15bn-on-unused-covid-supplies-watchdog-finds

63. Concern Over Corruption Red Flags In 20% Of UK's PPE Procurement. (2021, April 22). Transparency International UK. https://www.transparency.org.uk/track-and-trace-uk-PPE-procurement-corruption-risk-VIP-lane

64. Scott, R. (2024, November 14). More Than a Million Pallets of Unusable Covid PPE Costing £8 Billion Have So Far Gone Up in Smoke. Byline Times. https://bylinetimes.com/2024/11/14/more-than-a-million-pallets-of-unusable-covid-ppe-costing-8-billion-have-so-far-gone-up-in-smoke/

65. Supply Chain Coordination Limited. Letter dated 20 November 2024. reference SCCL-FOI-2024/25-121.

66. Supply Chain Coordination Limited. Letter dated 22 January 2025. reference SCCL-FOI-2024/25-134.

67. Ironmonger, J. (2024, June 25). Government writes off £1.4bn of PPE from Covid deal. BBC. https://www.bbc.co.uk/news/articles/cll476qzm85o

68. Supply Chain Coordination Limited. Letter dated 22 January 2025. reference SCCL-FOI-2024/25-134.

69. Ironmonger, J. (2024, June 25). Government writes off £1.4bn of PPE from Covid deal. BBC. https://www.bbc.co.uk/news/articles/cll476qzm85o

70. Davey, M. (2024, March 7). Fire near St Mary's Stadium: here is all we know so far. Daily Echo. https://www.dailyecho.co.uk/news/24168163.fire-near-st-marys-stadium-know-far/

71. Hampshire & Isle of Wight, Fire Investigation form. Incident VH040826 dated 06/03/2024. Obtained via Freedom of Information request.

72. Ironmonger, J. (2024, June 25). Government writes off £1.4bn of PPE from Covid deal. BBC. https://www.bbc.co.uk/news/articles/cll476qzm85o

Chapter 7: Held to account?

1. Structure Of The Inquiry – UK Covid-19 Inquiry. (n.d.). UK Covid-19 Inquiry. Retrieved May 17, 2024, from https://covid19.public-inquiry.uk/structure-of-the-inquiry/

2. Procurement (Module 5) – UK Covid-19 Inquiry. (n.d.). UK Covid-19

Inquiry. Retrieved May 17, 2024, from https://covid19.public-inquiry.uk/modules/procurement-module-5/

3. Module five Provisional Outline of Scope Procurement and distribution of key equipment and supplies. (n.d.). Covid19.Public-Inquiry.Uk. Retrieved May 17, 2024, from https://covid19.public-inquiry.uk/wp-content/uploads/2023/10/24092125/2023-09-28-M5-FINAL-Provisional-Outline-of-Scope-as-approved-by-Chair-28_09_2023.pdf

4. Scott, R. (2025, April 16). The Sheer Scale of the COVID 'VIP Lane' PPE Scandal Has Still Not Been Revealed Five Years On. *Byline Times*. https://bylinetimes.com/2025/04/16/covid-inquiry-vip-ppe/

5. Scott, R. (2025, April 2025). Company That Supplied Hundreds of Millions of Pounds of Unusable COVID Tests Saw Profits Skyrocket to £178 Million After Lobbying Conservative Peer for Contract. *Byline Times*. https://bylinetimes.com/2025/04/28/vip-covid-testing/

6. Scott, R. (2025, March 21). Civil Servants Felt Pressured Into Giving 'Special Treatment' to Conservative-Connected COVID PPE Suppliers. *Byline times*. https://bylinetimes.com/2025/03/21/covid-inquiry-vip-fast-lane/

7. Scott, R. (2025, April 11). Matt Hancock Intervened to Help Conservative Donor's Pizza Firm Land Lucrative Covid PPE Contract. *Byline Times*. https://bylinetimes.com/2025/04/11/matt-hancock-covid-ppe-vip/

8. Scott, R. (2025, March 07). Conservative Peer Lord Feldman Helped 'Good Friend' of Michael Gove Win VIP PPE Deal. *Byline Times*. https://bylinetimes.com/2025/03/07/conservative-peer-lord-feldman-helped-good-friend-of-michael-gove-win-vip-ppe-deal/

9. Scott, R. (2025, May 01). Private Correspondence Reveals How David Cameron Helped Old Etonian School Friend Fast-Track COVID Testing Firm. *Byline Times*. https://bylinetimes.com/2025/05/01/david-cameron-covid-vip-ppe/

10. REVIEW INTO THE DEVELOPMENT AND USE OF SUPPLY CHAIN FINANCE (AND ASSOCIATED SCHEMES) IN GOVERNMENT PART 2: RECOMMENDATIONS AND SUGGESTIONS. (2021, August 5). GOV.UK. https://assets.publishing.service.gov.uk/government/uploads/system/uploads/attachment_data/file/1018176/A_report_by_Nigel_Boardman_into_the_Development_and_Use_of_Supply_Chain_Finance__and_associated_schemes__related_to_Greensill_Capital_in_Government_-_Recommendations_and_Suggestions.pdf

11. Durrant, T. (2021, October). The Boardman review What the review into standards in public life got right – and what it missed. Institute for

Government. https://www.instituteforgovernment.org.uk/sites/default/files/publications/boardman-review.pdf

12. Boardman Review of Government Procurement in the COVID-19 pandemic one. Introduction and executive summary. (n.d.). GOV.UK. Retrieved May 17, 2024, from https://assets.publishing.service.gov.uk/media/60896ff0e90e076ab07a6d83/Boardman_Review_of_Government_COVID-19_Procurement_final_report.pdf

13. Beizsley, D. (2020, November 23). Government Must Get A Grip On Conflicts Of Interest In Public Procurement Or Risk Losing The UKs Reputation As A Fair Place To Do Business – Spotlight On Corruption. Spotlight On Corruption. https://www.spotlightcorruption.org/government-must-get-a-grip-on-conflicts-of-interest-in-public-procurement-or-risk-losing-the-uks-reputation-as-a-fair-place-to-do-business/

14. Track and Trace, Identifying corruption risks in UK public procurement for the Covid-19 Pandemic. (2021, April). Transparency International UK. https://www.transparency.org.uk/sites/default/files/pdf/publications/Track%20and%20Trace%20-%20Transparency%20International%20UK.pdf

15. COVID-19: Government procurement and supply of Personal Protective Equipment Forty-Second Report of Session 2019–21. (2021, February 4). House of Commons Public Accounts Committee. https://committees.parliament.uk/publications/4607/documents/46709/default/

16. The supply of personal protective equipment (PPE) during the COVID-19 pandemic. (2020, November 25). National Audit Office. https://www.nao.org.uk/wp-content/uploads/2020/11/The-supply-of-personal-protective-equipment-PPE-during-the-COVID-19-pandemic-Summary.pdf

Chapter 8. Afterword

1. Fraser, D. (2022, March 30). Covid-19: How much has it cost?. BBC. https://www.bbc.co.uk/news/uk-scotland-60924286

About the author

Russell Scott is a Yorkshire-based writer, journalist and former investigator at Good Law Project. During the pandemic he led Good Law Project's investigative work into corruption, unlocking democracy and environmental issues. His journalism has appeared in the *Guardian*, the BBC, the *Sunday Times*, the *Mirror*, *Byline Times* and many other publications. His investigative work was nominated for a British Journalism Award in 2019.

Russell was responsible for uncovering crucial details about the governments contracts for PPE, Covid testing equipment and ventilators during the pandemic and was responsible for successfully challenging the UK government to provide the names of the companies who benefited from the VIP lane.

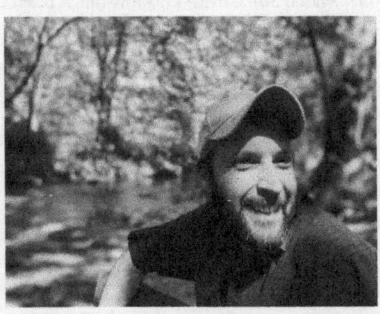